BLENDER ALCHEMY:

YOUR GUIDE TO CREATING DELICIOUS AND TRANSFORMATIVE ELIXIRS

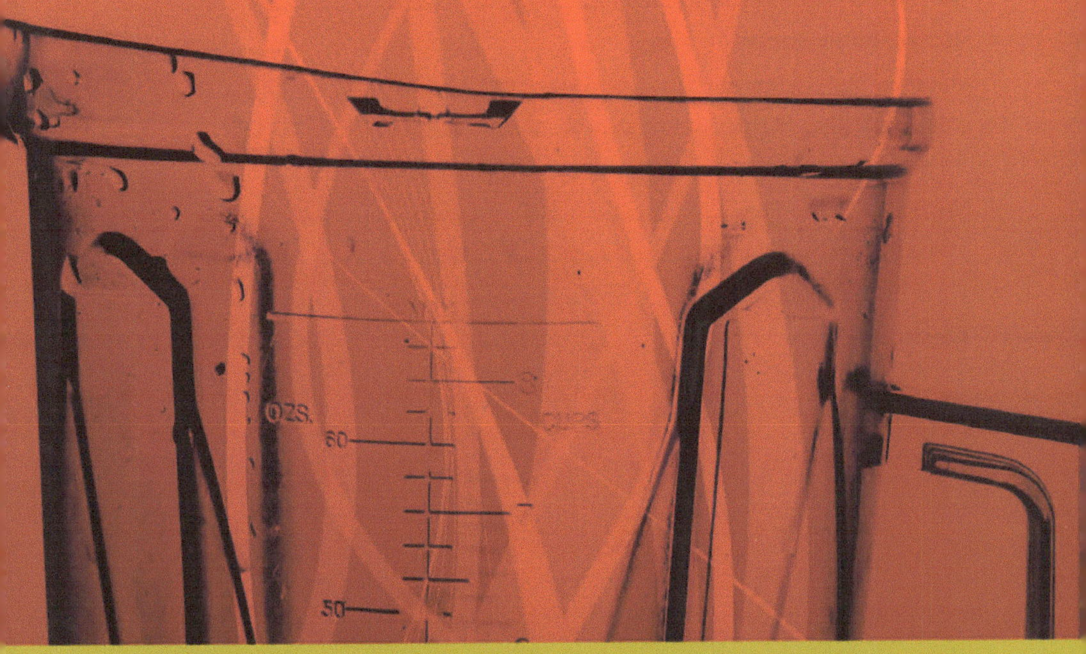

CREATED BY
BRANDON GILBERT

Table of Contents

My story and why I have created this book

I began making elixirs and consuming tonic herbs in early 2005, and it was truly love at first sight. While my first elixirs were nearly undrinkable, I knew there was something profound and worthy of deep exploration hidden within. Fueled by this initial inspiration, I have spent the last seven years tirelessly researching, experimenting, and refining my craft. This book represents the pinnacle of those countless hours and is a glimmering snapshot of where I am today.

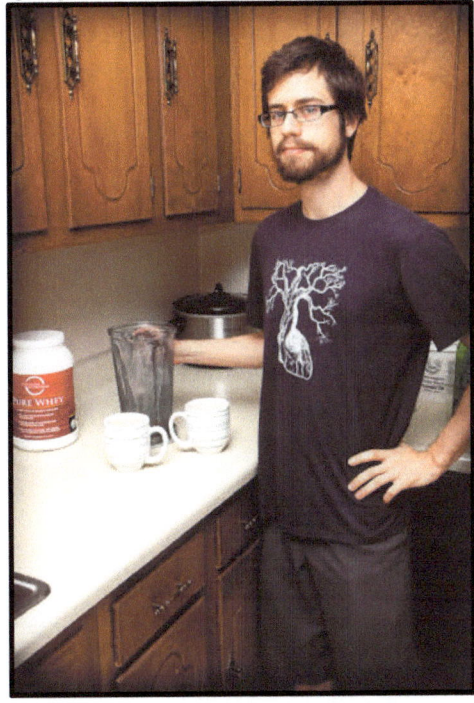

I wrote this book to distill my knowledge and experience into simple and easy-to-apply principles, which will allow you to leverage my experience. In short, this will save you a lot of time, energy, and money, and in essence, will hopefully allow you to avoid the mistakes that I have made along this path.

In late 2006, I was so inspired by elixirs and the transformative effects they had in my life that I decided to open a Tonic Elixir Bar here in Louisville, KY. This allowed me to essentially put all of my ideas, theories, and hypothesis to the test. I spent next two and half years making elixirs for the public for forty to sixty hours per week. If we were to do the math, that would be about one hundred weeks times forty, so where around four thousand hours of elixir-crafting. Keep in mind this is totally a low-ball rough estimate. During this time frame when I wasn't working the bar, I was lecturing and educating locally doing what I could to spread awareness about the transformative abilities of these potent elixirs and tonic herbs.

Somewhere in late 2008, I decided I wanted to reach out to more people and broaden my audience. This was the impetus that has led to where I am today. I saw that in order to reach more people, I would have to take everything online. That is exactly what I did in late 2009/early 2010 when I launched Hyperion TV and Hyperion Herbs.

It is now early 2012, and Hyperion Herbs and Hyperion TV have both matured from their first incarnations. Hyperion Herbs now has clients from all over the planet while Hyperion TV has well over eleven thousand subscribers. These achievements bring a smile to my face and fill me with contentment, but I feel as though I am just getting started.

We find ourselves at an interesting and profound time in history where in the fate of the planet is seemingly hanging by a delicate thread. Many of our brothers and sisters are plagued with illness and disease, whereas simultaneously, many are starting to wake up and seek alternatives to the shortcomings of the mainstream programs. Herein lies our collective challenge and opportunity, and in other words, where this all comes together.

The main goal and purpose of this book is to demystify and simplify the consumption and utilization of these powerful tonic substances. This is important because these things won't work if we don't eat them. We don't eat them if we don't like them. The challenge here is that due to our modern programming, these powerful foods are generally less than appealing to our taste buds. We must ask ourselves, how can adapt to this and overcome this hurdle?

The answer is elixirs.

Just how powerful is the most powerful herb if no one eats it?

About just as powerful as a bedtime story.

Elixirs allow us to get these tenacious substances into our bodies in a way that is familiar and delicious. This allows the bodies' programmed resistance to be put aside so that these foods can come in and work the magic they were created for. Thus, a benevolent cycle is begun. We accomplish this by leveraging the basic understanding that we as humans crave things that are tasty to our palate, and secondly, that our body will crave things which it feels to be nourishing. These two components joined together form a powerful synergy that can open doors for massive transformation in the body.

To sum it up, I wrote this book to share with you my years of experience and knowledge, as you open the doors for massive transformations and upgrades.

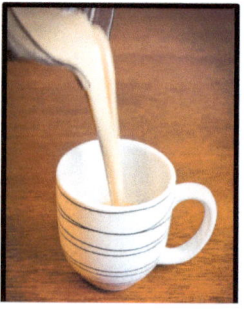 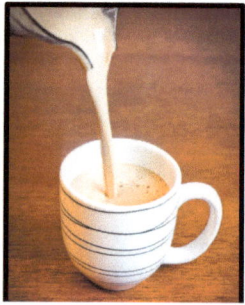 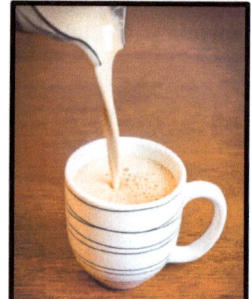

What Is An Elixir?

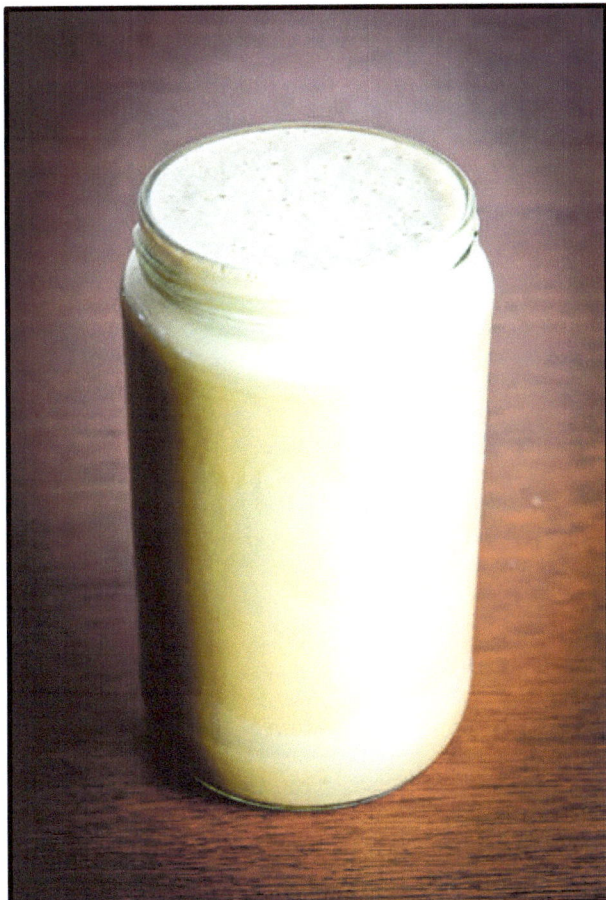

An elixir is generally a tea or other liquid that has been transformed into a food, or a meal, due to the addition of fat, carbohydrates, and protein.

So basically the equation for an elixir is:

elixir = tea + calories (fats, carbs, protein)

This combination turns a medicine into food and food into medicine.

Elixirs serve as a delivery vehicle for all of the herbs and superfoods that one may decide to ingest.

Elixirs can be a personalized, fine-tuned, and intelligently crafted medicinal food.
Gone are the days of "the kitchen sink" smoothie. Elixirs are a more elegant, intelligent, evolved, and effective form of nutrition.

Like Hippocrates, the founder of modern medicine said:
"Let food be thy medicine, and medicine thy food."

Yet, never before has it been easier to fully actualize the meaning and intention behind that statement.

Elixirs are by far the quickest, easiest, and most potent method to realize and embody this teaching.

I wonder if Hippocrates knew that one day there would be thousands of us living by this axiom and transforming it into such a beautiful and elegant art and science.

Either way, we owe much to the ancient herbalist, healers, and alchemists who really paved the way and opened the doors of knowledge for us. Out of gratitude, we take this ancient art and science to a more modern and evolved level.

Elixirs can allow us to eat less. If I'm out on the go, or running out with little to no time, to actually have to eat a meal is hard to come by. Rather than just crashing blood sugar or eating a bunch of little snacks, I can just have a drink. I can sip on it and keep my energy sustained, while also keeping my calorie levels adequate. I'll feel great and not so bogged down from either not eating or eating a fast, nutrient-poor or unbalancing snack. Elixirs are actually more absorbable and digestible than solid foods because they're in that liquid state. The ingredients are easier on the body and in turn, our organs can rest. As we are still getting the calories, we're still getting sustainable nutrition. In this respect, we really don't have to eat as much, taking a burden off of at least one meal a day. You don't have to make the process a big ordeal. All it takes is five minutes throwing things in the blender and blending it up. Once you put it in your jar, you're out the door, and you have your meal for the next three to four hours. The convenience of elixirs is one of its greatest benefits, taking fast food to an even faster plane with outlandishly higher nutritional content.

Elixirs have even been held in high regard throughout history. If you go back through time, the word "elixir" reveals itself in various places and times, and was most often used to reference a medicinal beverage used to cure ailments or that of a dignified purpose. There has always been the elixir of immortality, or the ultimate elixir, that has been sought after by many cultures. The formulations and substances that have been considered elixirs have been lost in modern times because we thought, "Oh, that stuff is weird and mystical and it definitely doesn't work." Alas, we have recently excavated this term with definitive ground, and using our blender and all of our technology, we can craft our own and be our own alchemist/healer/shaman/herbalist in the privacy of our own home, for ourselves, for our friends and family, in a way that makes sense to us.

Making myself a specific fine-tuned elixir on a regular basis is one of the most transformational activities I've added into my lifestyle thus far. Having made my daily grail, I insure that I have started the day off on the right foot, with positive energy and momentum in the right direction. Whether you didn't sleep the night before and need to work all day, are trying to build up muster for your work out, need extra focus for a test, or just seeking your daily wake up call, you can supplement with sustainable energy without the crash with a well-made, self-tuned elixir.

How To Be An Elixir Master

Elixirs are quintessentially the easiest and the quickest way to incorporate all of the powerful herbs that are out there, all the amazing supplements and powders, nutrient-rich proteins, and all the superfoods that are out there. You're able to put it all together into something that tastes good, is quick and easy to make, and makes you feel amazing. On top of that, it's custom made and fine tuned just for you. It's not something you go to the store and get off the shelf, which is more or less what someone else says your body needs. It allows you to tune into your own intuition, to your own gut, and ask yourself, what do I need, what is appropriate, what is the best thing for me to take right now?

Elixirs allow us to make something that is completely customized and adapted to our individual needs. Because I am different, my physiology and my emotions and my whole system are different from yours and yours are different from your next-door neighbors, etc. Also, understand we all deal with different things, so for me to say, "Here's exactly what you should do", to a degree, that could be helpful and important, but it is also limiting. If I'm sitting on a computer for 8 hours a day, and you're riding a bike for 8 hours a day, we're going to need different substances for our body. If you're dealing with lower back and knee pain, you're going to need a different approach than someone who is dealing with chronic autoimmune conditions.

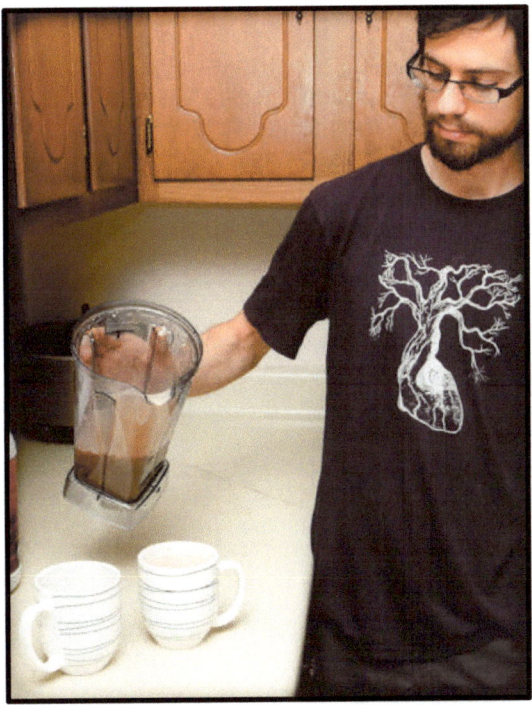

I highly suggest and recommend that whenever you're crafting an elixir, to really have an end result in mind. To have a purpose, a vision, or a mission for the elixir will truly allow the formula to emerge. This is a mindset and a strategy that you need to have in place that will then allow you to craft the perfect drink, the perfect elixir for yourself, no matter what your ingredients are, and no matter what situation you're in.

You figure out a little bit about what works with what and how they go together. It's very similar to cooking. You learn what has friends and what balances what. It is a very intuitive and personalized process, as it's more artistic than scientific.

The first thing that we need to understand is what is the perfect elixir and how to define such a term? To me, the perfect elixir is making the appropriate drink for you in that moment. Meaning, it is satiating and it is something that is not going to pick you up and then drop you off. It means it is something that would be able to sustain you, balance your metabolism, balance your energy, and feed you for an extended period of time.

There are several questions you can ask yourself when starting with an end result in mind such as, Is this something I'm just making as a quick snack? Is this something

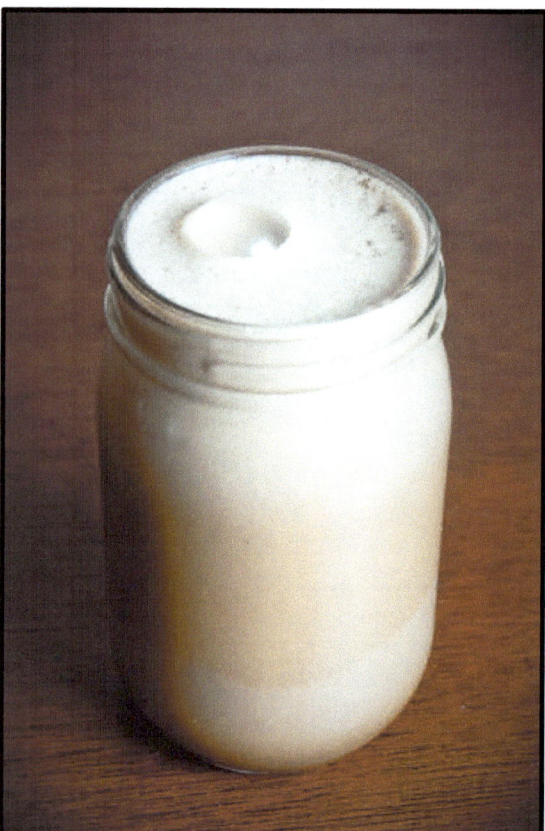

that's going to need to be a meal? If so, how long do I need to be sustained for? What flavors am I craving? How am I feeling right now? How can my elixir aid in orienting me for what I am about to do?

All of these things need to be in the back of your mind and need to be answered, and then you can make it happen.

The next step in becoming an elixir master is contingent upon your metabolism. What I mean by that is, by knowing whether you burn carbohydrates or fats or proteins as your primary source of fuel. Now, most people are going to burn fat and protein, or some balance of both, and very small amount of people are actually going to be those who burn carbs the best. I can tell you, from my years of making elixirs and drinks, both for myself at home and for the public at my bar, that people are very sensitive to high ups and even lower lows. If a drink is not well balanced, it can affect your blood sugar or leave you hungry and exhausted, so making a drink that's tuned up to you metabolism is huge for you elixir art.

That's the main thing to making the perfect elixir- to understand your metabolism and understand what you burn best. With that, consciously and intelligently choose the majority of your drink. Then, adding your herbs and other things, fine tuning it based on what your intention is. Whether that's to build your immune system, build your jing, nourish your spleen chi, or just a protein drink or a meal. Simply having the idea of what you specifically have in mind, and not try to do it all in once.

The only problem here is that there can be a tremendous learning curve on how to put these things together and what the appropriate amounts to ensure they taste good and make you feel good, without making you sick or inhibiting loss of expensive product. And I can say, personally, I have made so many mistakes, wasted so many expensive ingredients, and made myself sick on many occasions from just overdosing on certain things. But at the end, I came out learning what not to do and what to do and how to do it, when to do it, how often, how to combine it, etc.

This is exactly what this book helps you to avoid, and instead, cut straight to the most delicious and transformative results you set out for.

The Biggest Mistakes People Make When Creating Elixirs:

We live in a really exciting and unique time because we can have access to all these amazing herbs, super foods, and crazy amazing fats and oils and sweeteners, and spices and everything from all of history. We have the best of every single culture that has existed at the tips of our fingers. We have it all, so okay, what am I going to do with it?

In this section we are going to talk about one of the biggest mistakes that I see people making when creating elixirs. This applies to whether it's for yourself at home or whether it's in a retail environment that you're buying for generally really high prices. I've learned the pitfalls of elixir-making the hard way, and I hope to save you all the trouble and fun aches I've experienced in my elixirs, and at times, mad-scientist experiments.

The first, and possibly one of the biggest problems I ran into was not creating sustainable energy with my drinks. I'd make something that tasted divine, at least in my opinion at the time, yet an hour later I'd be fatigued or hungry. For a while, this had been the case, and I realized it's one of the easiest mistakes to make when making "health" beverages.

What I was doing was not putting enough protein and fat into my drinks, and instead, putting in way too much sugar, whether it was agave, honey, healthy fruits, or whatever it was. I've now learned to add a lot more protein, and moderate amounts of fat, and then just a little stevia and maybe a little bit of honey or coconut sugar just to balance or reveal certain flavors. For most people that are making drinks, fruits, sweeteners and milks are the base, making it very not only very sweet, but high in sugar. So really we want to let go of that and move away from that old paradigm and replace it with this new version of actually understanding ourselves and taking a second to ask ourselves, what's our primary source of fuel and what's going to be the best choice? For most people, that's going to be a combination of protein and fat and minimal amounts of sugar. It's usually best to avoid most sugars and stick with stevia, raw honey, or unrefined and raw forms of sugars, and as fruit is beneficial in some ways, it is essentially just another form of sugar. This mistake can often incept the next biggest elixir no-no.

Once its highly sweetened, one may begin to feel safe to add the herbs, and maybe a little of this and a little of that. The reality is, it's not really sustaining and it's still based on the old paradigm of, I've got frozen bananas, blueberries, and milk, lets dump it all in the blender with every herb and spice I own and that's going to be my daily drink.

The biggest mistake is overkill on ingredients. Too many ingredients and too broad of a focus usually causes indigestion, gas, bloating, tiredness, headaches, diarrhea, or whatever other symptom that may manifest. It is really indicating an imbalance and a poor level of craftsmanship, if in a retail environment, as well as misunderstanding of the metabolism.

On top of all of that, it could be just too many flavors.

If you are just stacking mesquite and vanilla bean, and then you add a little cinnamon, a little agave, a little honey, and a little stevia, and then you add in five herbs, a bunch of coconut oil, and a bunch of protein powders. All of those flavors and ingredients could easily be overwhelming to both your body and your taste buds. Essentially, you body is being pulled in all of these different directions and won't know how to digest and make these ingredients useful.

Within this mistake, I'd like to address the action of using too many different herbs or "medicinal" ingredients.

On one hand you could have a very stimulating herb, then you have a calming herb, to which then you could have just used one adaptogenic herb, but you used all three anyway, along with ten other sprinkles of the luring herbal kingdom you've worked so hard to establish. As tempting as it may be, you could find yourself wanting to throw five different herbs in your drink, which are pulling the body in all these weird directions. This typically causes indigestion and thus, undermines the results for the person who actually consumes the elixir, and becomes a huge waste of money.

One reason this is happening is because we are really lucky right now, and we have tons of ingredients that are appealing, taste good, fun, and that make us feel great, and sometimes we just want to throw them all in. I totally understand and relate to, because I did that for so many years and wasted a lot of money, upset my stomach, gave myself a lot of indigestion and probably sometimes did more harm than good. It's important to really just simplify and simplify again to keep things at a peak functional level.

Sometimes less is more.

For that reason, again, I must reiterate it is important to start with the end in mind. Starting off with wide eyes will leave you wide open for unforeseen side effects that are generally not associated with any of the ingredients you actually used. If you begin making your elixir, asking yourself the questions we reviewed in the previous section, avoiding the elixir-killers above, you will not only be able to quickly learn how certain ingredients can synergize, but also how they can positively comply with your specific metabolism.

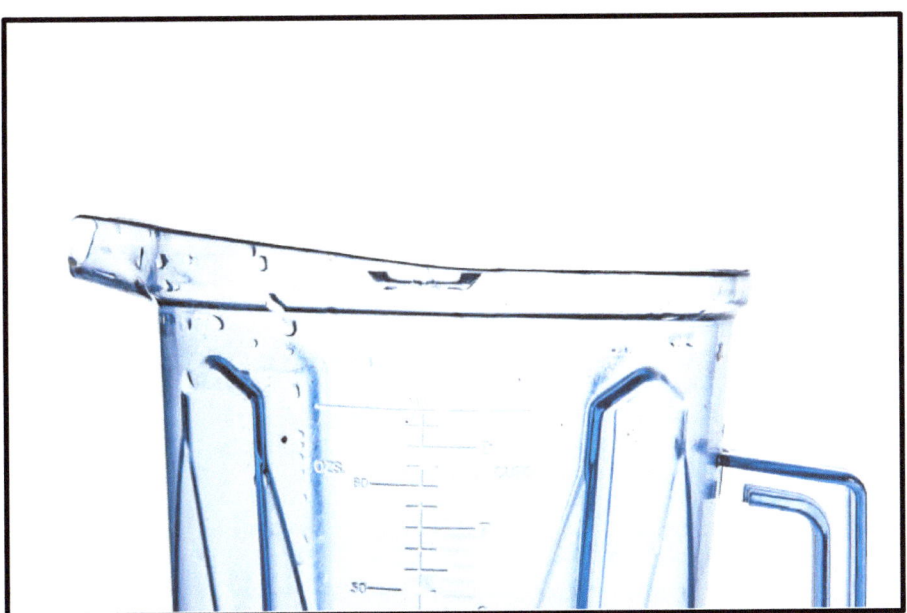

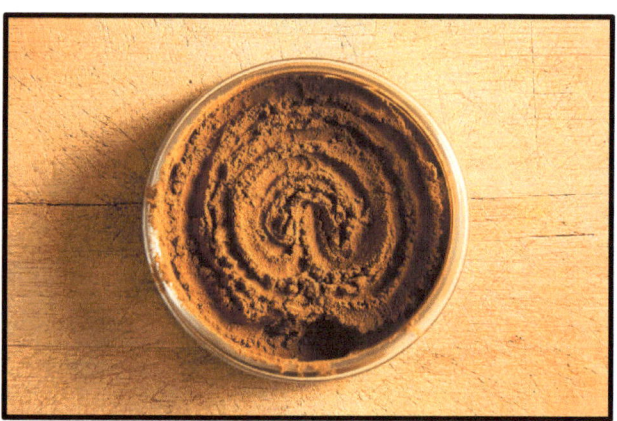

Why Take Tonic Herbs?

Tonic herbs have profound anti-inflammatory and antioxidant effect on the body, which, in my opinion, is always a good thing. The tonics like reishi, gynostemma, and cordyceps are profound at protecting the body from oxidation- cellular oxidation, and lipid oxidation- meaning preventing the fats in our body from oxidizing, which is really strongly correlated to the aging and breaking down process. If you look at a car rusting, that's the oxidation process. That's the process of that metal being broken down. The oxidation process in our body is a very similar process. The more we can stop, prevent, and protect against it, the better off we'll be. Life itself can be pretty inflammatory, as far as allergies from foods, things in the air and water, and in our clothes. These can all stimulate an inflammatory response in the body, as tonic herbs can help to cool them down, retiring that impeding issue from your bodily processes.

Tonic herbs also protect your body by balancing, strengthening, and tonifying the immune system. Not stimulating or depressing, but balancing and strengthening. Basically, what they can do is enter your body, sense deficiencies, sense excesses, and balance, so that we're not dealing with an imbalanced immune system. They then rally up all our natural killer cells, macrophages, and lymphocytes. They can get them going and say, "Hey, go out, do your job! Time to clean house!" All of these functions work together to diminish viral, bacterial, and fungal deposits in the body. Conditions such as allergies, little rashes, and other symptoms that surface are basically related to the immune system, indicative of imbalances and latent processes. Those can all be knocked out from the source.

The following facet of herbs is less physical, as it delves into a little more etheric, energetic, or spiritual part of your being. Herbs like reishi, schizandra, and gynostemma can work on our spirit and consciousness. Reishi is actually called "The Great Protector" because it strengthens our "wei chi," which is our chi that is generated by our body. It's kind of like our protective aura, or our protective shield that we radiate. If that is charged strong enough, it can repel both physical and non-physical deviations from entering into our perception field. I have learned this through both my experience with reishi and many other people who have shared a similar experience. As short-term effects may include increased positivity and mood-shifts, there are more long-term, as well as permanent benefits, such as helping you deal with negative thought patterns, release those negative thought patterns, and work through old things that could be attracting even more new negativity to you. That is certainly as brief as it can get, but you get the idea.

Those are just three of the many ways that the tonic herbs are protective- they're massive anti-inflammatory antioxidants to our body, they are immune-modulating, and they help to protect us from negativity by assisting in creating a stronger protective shield.

Why is it now that these tonic herbs are really coming out and coming up to the forefront of a historical and chronological context?

People have used them for thousands of years, so why are they gaining popularity now in this point in history?

Basically, right now seems to be one of the most toxic times to be alive on the planet, in regards to pollution of the environment, chemicals, air, water, food, etc. Even our clothes and sheets are both made from and most often washed in synthetic chemicals that are releasing themselves into our bodies all the time. We're driving in cars, breathing in car exhaust, as we keep the windows rolled up. We hang out in small places where people are smoking cigarettes, or sitting inside all day, staring at electronic screens, surrounded by WiFi connections or EMFs, as the list goes on and on and on. Though this may induce a grim outlook on the world and threaten our given time to be alive, it is our responsibility to take our lives into our own hands and use the resources that have been time-tested and re-gifted, just for us.

So sure, things are getting kind of chaotic right now, but the universe remains in balance, so for the people who are open and receptive, the tools to adapt and the tools to stay safe and protected are being presented. In my opinion, tonic herbs stand at the front of the line of the army of resources that are coming into our consciousness (and rescue) right now in this point in history.

I find tonic herbs to be a staple for our health, as they're so important to be consuming on a daily basis to protect us from this inevitable circulation of harmful and environmental aggravations. They serve to fill in our gaps, to nourish our deficiencies, to calm our excesses, to restore balance of homeostasis, and to take us to higher levels of health, consciousness and vitality, all of which we were meant to have.

About The Ingredients

Astragalus Extract

Astragalus is known primarily as tonic to the Chi and Triple Warmer systems in Chinese medicine. What this means is that it's a great tonic to the respiratory, immune, digestive, and metabolic functions in the body. Astragalus is being heavily researched for its anti-aging and longevity properties, as well. One chemical in particular known as astragaloside IV has been shown to assist in DNA repair and is thus believed to be a great aid in combatting the process of aging. I, personally, like to use it primarily for its great taste and its athletic enhancing properties.

Bentonite Clay

It might sound weird at first to eat clay, but it's been proven that most animals in nature intuitively eat it. This is because they know that clay absorbs poisons and toxins, which they are accumulating from their diet of wild plants. Wild plants typically contain alkaloids, which become toxic in larger quantities, thus animals eat the clay to absorb these toxins and mitigate the negative effects. It's also worth mentioning that many animals consume clay whenever they are getting sick or have ingested a pathogenic organism. What we can learn from this is that clay is a useful tool and ally to easily detoxify and cleanse our bodies. This is important because we are constantly being exposed to toxins in our environment, which if not efficiently eliminated, will gradually accumulate in the body.

Black Pepper

Black pepper is a really common and widely used spice, but most people don't realize that it can actually have quite medicinal effects. I use it to enhance and potentiate the effects of herbs, as well as aiding in digestion, but again quality matters, as not all black pepper will have the same effects.

BrainOn Flakes

BrainON is one of my favorite supplements of all time because it's stands as a gift that keeps on giving. The product itself is actually an extract of Blue Green Algae and is extremely rich in the psychoactive compound known as PEA. PEA greatly increases creativity, concentration, focus, and it also induces a wonderful natural high, as I can personally vouch for all of these accounts. On top of that it contains many potent antioxidants and neurotransmitter modulating agents, which synergize and enhance the actions of PEA. BrainOn is also very rich in chlorophyll, minerals, and amino acids.

Blue Majik Powder

This is also an extract of algae, but instead, comes from Spirulina. It's actually the blue pigment from these algae and is rich in the compound, Phycocyanin. The powder itself is an amazing bright blue color and I highly recommend you check it out and truly experience how the color speaks for itself. Phycoyanin has been shown to be a potent anti-inflammatory by inhibiting COX-2 while also enhancing anti-oxidant production. It has also been shown to stimulate bone marrow and stem cell production. This is really a powerful, effective substance, which we are extremely lucky to have access to.

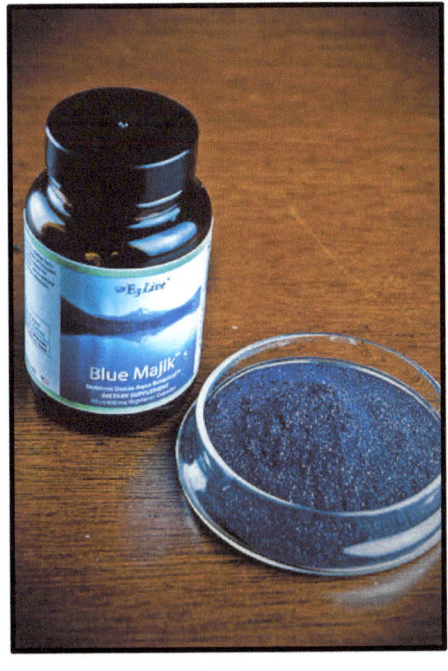

Cacao Powder

Raw Cacao Powder is one of the most popular raw food/superfood products on the market today. Quality matters and not all raw cacao powders are created equal. Please see the resources section to learn more about some good sources. I like to use cacao because, well, lets face it, it is DELICIOUS and can make any elixir into a decadent experience. Nutritionally raw cacao powder is rich in antioxidants, minerals, as well as many unique psychoactive compounds like anandamide and PEA.

Camu Camu

Camu is a berry that comes from the rain forest and is most well known as the highest source of Vitamin C on the planet. This is primarily what attracts me to this herb, as this potent dose of Vitamin C is great for the immune system and for enhancing detoxification. Also it helps to synergize and potentiate many of the herbs used in these elixir recipes, as Vitamin C helps to make most tonic herbs for absorbable and useful in your body.

Cardamom

I like to use cardamom for its carminative and digestive supporting effects. This is a very potent and fragrant herb, so a little goes a long way. However, it is quite delicious so a pinch is really all you need.

Cinnamon

Cinnamon is, hands down, one of the most popular and delicious herbs on the planet. But again, quality matters, and not all cinnamon is created equal. This herb has been known to balance blood sugar and aid in digestion. However, the caveat here is that only True Cinnamon or Ceylon Cinnamon has these benefits. Please see the resources section to see where you can get the real stuff. If you've never had, then I HIGHLY recommend you try it and see what cinnamon is really all about. The real stuff tastes so good you can eat it right from the bag, strikingly similar to the taste of the classic Red Hots Candy.

Cloves

I like to use clove for its carminative and digestive supporting effects. It's also known to be great for the immune system, given its anti-viral and anti-parasitic properties. This is a very potent herb, so a little goes a long way. However, it is quite delicious, so a pinch is really all you need, as it will radiate its glory into your whole drink.

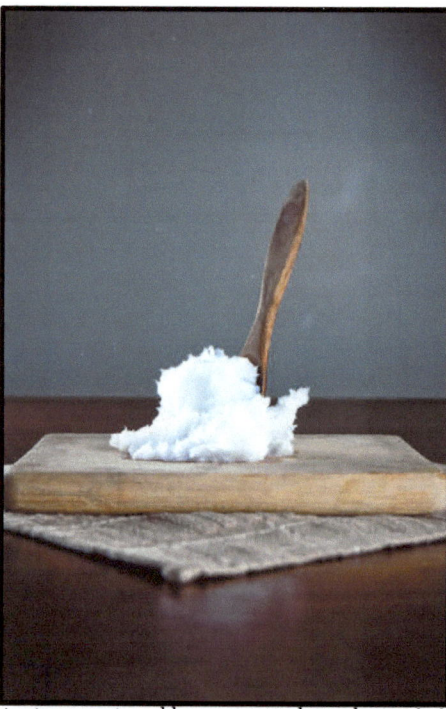

Coconut Oil

Coconut Oil is one of the most nutritious and delicious oil available today. It's my favorite oil to cook with, to put in elixirs, and to use on my skin. It is a deeply nourishing food, both internally and externally, and is something that is pretty well tolerated by most people. Don't be confused by the fact that it is fat. Fat is an ESSENTIAL part of the diet. The bottom line is quality matters, and not all fats are created equal. Coconut oil provides fat that is easy to digest and that actually supports weight loss and raises energy levels.

Coconut Crystals

This is, by FAR, my favorite sweetener of all time. It is made from the sap of the coconut tree, and is abundant in 17 Amino Acids, B Vitamins, Vitamin C, as well as FOS, which is a pre-biotic that supports gut health. On top of that, it tastes great and has a pretty low glycemic index of 35.

Colostrum Powder

Colostrum is known as the first milk or 6-hour milk because all mammals produce it 6 hours before and after birth. It is the most nourishing substance for the newborn because it provides pretty much every known nutrient, immune factor, growth factors, and probiotic. It is also used to educate and inform the newborn's immune system. Basically, the mother downloads all of her immune information into the newborn so that it can safely adapt and survive in the environment. Because it can provide similar effects to us, we consume it as a dietary supplement. Quality matters here and you need to be sure you are dealing with a legitimate and high integrity company that only takes the colostrum that the calf doesn't consume. I recommend Surthrival, as they have the best colostrum on the market.

Cordyceps Extract

This is actually one of, if not the most, expensive commodities on the planet right now. Of course, I am referring to the wild specimens, which come from Tibet and parts of China. Luckily, we are able to access cultivated varieties at a fraction of the cost. The good news is that many of the cultivated varieties have been shown to be more potent than the wild stuff. Many studies have shown that many of the cultivated strains actually have a richer concentration in the known active constituents.

I like to use cordyceps primarily for its jing building and athletic enhancing properties. It directly nourishes both yin and yang jing energies while also tonifying the chi production from the lungs and spleen. It's also quite famous for its anti-inflammatory, anti-allergy, and immuno-balancing properties.

Dandelion Root

Dandelion root is similar to yellow dock they really get the liver going and in that light, are great to work with in the springtime. Dandelion root is used to stimulate bile production and liver detoxification. It's also a blood purifier and a mild laxative and diuretic. These properties are extra useful when stimulating detoxification in the liver, as they help escort toxins from the body in an efficient manner. For these reasons its great for short term cleansing, but obviously not ideal for long term, daily usage.

Ginger

Ginger is one the most famous, well known, and widely used herbs on the planet. It's mostly used for flavoring, but it actually has great medicinal effects. I use it mainly as a carminative or a digestive aid in recipes. It seems to aid in digestion, ease inflammation, and also boost and potentiate other herbs.

Gynostemma Tea

I consider gynostemma to be the most potent adaptogen on the planet. I say this because it contains the richest concentration of the adaptogenic saponins of any plant ever discovered. On top of that, it tastes great, is extremely affordable, and is easy to use. It is my favorite base for any elixir because it has such cohesive and balancing effect on the whole recipe. It seems to round things out, balance the effects, and soften any hard edges that a recipe might have.

He Shou Wu Extract

He Shou Wu has been classically regarded as one of the greatest anti-aging, rejuvenation, and longevity herbs in Chinese Medicine. He Shou Wu is classified as a tonic to the Kidney Yin Jing as well as to the blood. It's also said to have a stabilizing and grounded effect to the heart and nervous system, and it's for these reasons that many experience a calm sense of uplifted-ness after consuming this revered tonic herb. It's also extremely rich in

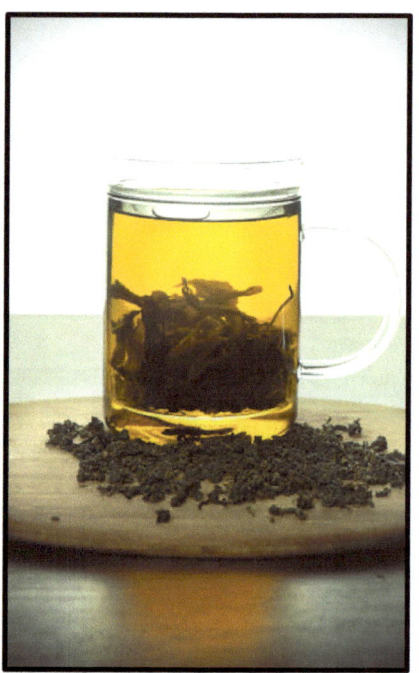

zinc and iron, which contributes to its tonic effects on the reproductive, immune, and nervous systems.

Kombucha

Kombucha is actually a colony of symbiotic yeast and bacteria. It is loaded with enzymes, probiotics, vitamins, and special acids, which aid in detoxification and digestion. Many people become hopelessly addicted to this because it is so delicious, nutritious, and fun to drink. To me it is truly one of the greatest beverages of all time, and I am a hopeless addict. Due to its concentration of enzymes and probiotics, kombucha is a great aid to digestion before, during, and after a meal.

Lemon Juice

Lemon juice is simply one of the best foods for the liver and gallbladder. In Chinese Medicine, the sour taste is said to stimulate to liver energy, I believe this provides some explanation as to why this food has such a beneficial effect on these organs. Lemon juice not only helps to stimulate bile flow, but it is quite beneficial for aiding and stimulating overall digestion and elimination. Lastly, lemon juice also helps to break up phlegm and calcification in the body, promoting circulation.

Mucuna Extract

Mucuna Pruriens comes from the Ayurvedic herbal system and is used as a tonic to the nervous, reproductive, and endocrine system. Modern research has revealed that mucuna contains a wide variety of psychoactive substances. The most famous of which is L-Dopa, which is the amino acid precursor to dopamine. Thus, mucuna can naturally boost and replenish our dopamine levels. Low levels of dopamine have been linked to a myriad of mental, emotional, and physical imbalances and it is for this reason that mucuna is becoming increasingly more famous and well known.

Polyrachis Extract

Polyrachis is, in my opinion, the ultimate jing building substance. And yes, it is actually an extract of ants. But not just any kind of ant, as it is a specific species that has been used in China as a food and medicine for hundreds, if not thousands, of years. Scientific research has also been done on this herb and confirmed the ancient claims. Aside from nourishing the jing energy, polyrachis provides the body with usable ATP, or adenosine triphosphate, which essentially translates to natural energy without any stimulation or crash.

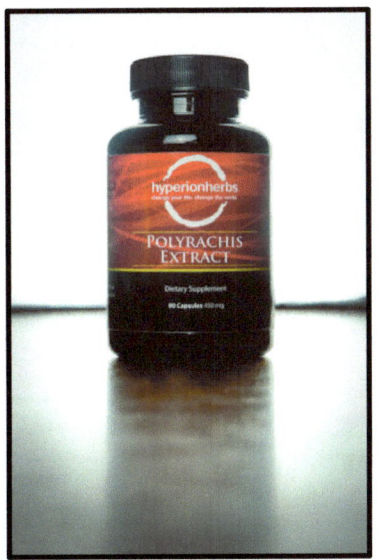

Reishi Extract

Reishi Mushroom is has been called "The Mushroom of Immortality" for at least one thousand years, and also happens to be the most scientifically researched and validated herb in history. I think those two criteria can speak for the magnitude of this herb. I use it primarily for enhancing the immune system, the liver, and also building the shen. Shen is one of the Three Treasures and translates as spirit. Reishi has a unique ability to help nurture our spirit and grow our consciousness. This is why many people turn to it for its anti-depression and anti-stress effects. This is actually what first attracted me to this herb. I had heard that it was used by Taoist monks for building spiritual energy and was hooked from that moment on.

Schizandra Juice

This is truly one of the greatest gifts of the herbal world. Simply put, this herb almost does it all. Its main uses for me are for benefiting the liver and also enhancing the mental functions. Schizandra is one of the best, if not the best, at cleansing the liver. It activates stage 1 and stage 2 detoxification. This is truly a unique quality and I do not know of another herb that is capable of this. Basically, what that translates to is that schizandra stimulates the liver to release a toxin, and most importantly, it then helps to safely escort the toxin from the body via the urine and feces. Many herbs stimulate the liver, Stage 1, but few actually stimulate the safe removal simultaneously, Stage 2. For mental and cognitive functions, schizandra is unsurpassed in its ability to enhance concentration, focus, learning, memory, and endurance. Studies have shown that it can improve all of the functions all the while calming and relaxing the nervous system. That is just two of my favorite fuctions out of the many that schizandra is capable. With all 5 flavors, it contains access to all 5 spirits, 12 meridians, and all 3 treasures, opening the doors to a well-rounded, full-sensory experience for both your taste buds and your body.

Stevia Extract
Stevia has been used as an herb for centuries by many indigenous cultures that referred to the herb as the sweet leaf or honey leaf. The plant came to the attention of the rest of the world when South American naturalist, Bertoni, "discovered" the plant in the late 1800's. After his report, the herb became widely used by herbalists in Paraguay. Stevia's most obvious and notable characteristic is its sweet taste. However, the sweet taste is not due to carbohydrate-based molecules, but to several non-caloric molecules called glycosides. Individuals who cannot tolerate sugar or other sweeteners can use stevia. The first glycoside molecule was isolated from stevia in 1931 by two French chemists named Bridel and Lavieille and called "Stevioside." During WWII, sugar shortages prompted England to begin investigation of stevia for use as a sweetener. Cultivation began under the direction of the Royal Botanical Gardens at Kew, but the project was abandoned in the aftermath of the war. It is the most delicious and healthy alternative to any sweetener.

Vanilla Powder
Vanilla is the second most expensive spice in the world, as growing vanilla commercially is an extremely labor intensive and delicate operation. This herb comes from the fruit of the orchid variety Vanilla Planifolia and is rich in the natural organic compound called vanillin. Along with more than a hundred other organic compounds, vanillin contributes to its unique flavor profile. Vanilla has long been purported to act as an aphrodisiac. In the 1700's, it was recommended by physicians to be consumed as an infusion or tincture for the purposes of male potency. An article written by the German physician in 1762 claimed that 342 impotent men were changed into astonishing lovers from drinking vanilla decoctions.

Whey Protein
Whey Protein helps to increase glutathione production, boost and regulate immune function, quickly refuel amino acid pools after an anabolic workout, and even be used as an easy meal replacement, all without stimulating a blood sugar spike. Plus it tastes GREAT and really adds an essential, milky, and basic element to any elixir.

Yellow Dock Root

Yellow dock is another herb I like to work with around springtime when I feel the need to really get the liver going. This is because in Chinese Medicine Spring is associated with the wood element and the liver. Yellow dock is used to stimulate bile production and liver detoxification. It's also a blood purifier and a mild laxative and diuretic. These properties are extra useful when stimulating detoxification in the liver as they help escort toxins from the body in an efficient manner. For these reasons its great for short term cleansing, but obviously not ideal for long term, daily usage.

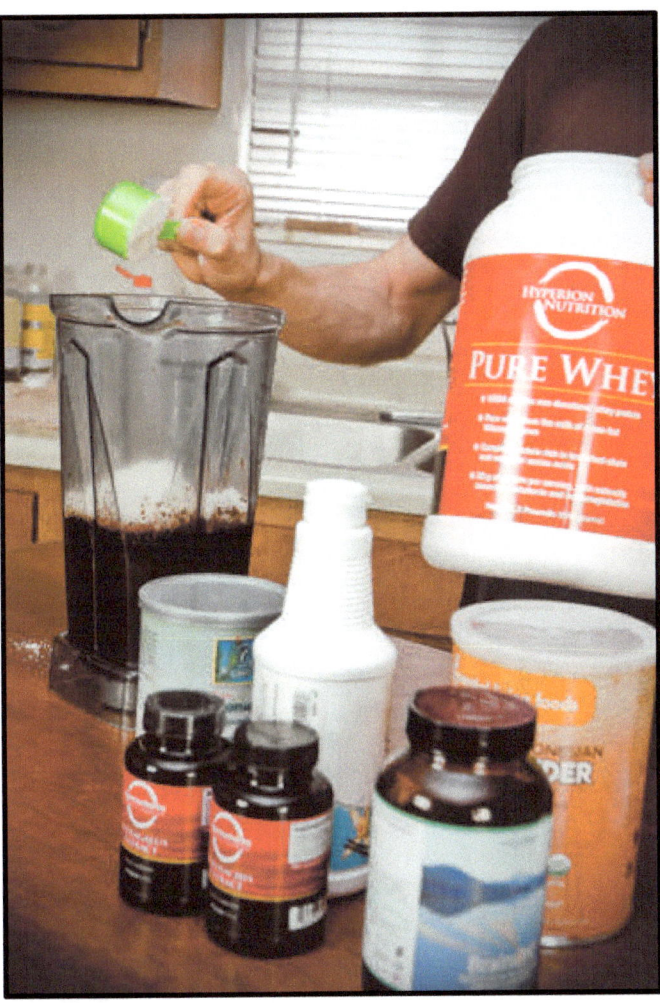

Supreme Athletic Elixir

This elixir is great to power up and get moving before a work out and also a great aid to recovery post work out. The herbs in this recipe are all highly regarded adaptogens that help the body handle stress and recover from stress much more effectively and efficiently. This is important for obvious reasons given the stress that exercise can put on the body. Gynostemma specifically does a few crucial things in that category. First, it helps the heart to pump blood more effectively and secondly, it helps to naturally boost nitric oxide production. Both of these are key elements for having proper blood circulation to make sure the nutrients are transported and the wastes are eliminated from the body.

Cordyceps and Polyrachis Ant are also great herbs that help us adapt to stress. In addition, both of these herbs naturally stimulate the production of ATP, or Adenosine Triphosate. If you don't know what that is, it is essentially the energy currency of our cells, and is the energy of our body. So for this reason, these herbs are particularly magical in their effects because they naturally help our bodies to have more energy, without any stimulation, side effect, or crash. This is totally a game-changer for the work out world given the popularly of stimulants of all kinds that are used to get one energized for a work out. Cordyceps also increases respiration and oxygen utilization by up to 30%-40%, depending on the study you read. This coupled with its ability to naturally boost ATP makes it an absolute superstar for increased energy, endurance, performance, strength, and recovery.

Astragalus is likely one of the most popular,well tolerated, and effective chi tonics. Now as we begin, I want to distinguish and make clear that when I mean chi and energy, I don't mean stimulation. I don't mean a jolt or a rush of energy that we often associate with the term "energy" or "energy tonic." Astragalus is something you can take at night before you go to bed or at any time, and it's not going to give you push you over the edge or impede natural function. When people think energy, we think coffee; we think Red Bull, or whatever, so I just want to make clear that astragalus doesn't act like this. It actually does not even act on the nervous system, stimulate the adrenals, or irritate at the body in any way. It produces more energy in the body at the fundamental level by toning up the basic cellular processes that generate our "true" energy.

The other ingredients are massively supportive and carefully chosen for this recipe, as well. Coconut oil is one of the easiest fats to digest and the fats it provides are not stored in the body, but instead are immediately converted into caloric energy. These kinds of calories lead to a longer, slower metabolic burn, thus equaling longer, more sustained energy and blood sugar levels. Coconut oil also adds amazing texture and truly supports the cohesion of the whole drink.

The coconut crystals are a great natural sweetener and are actually pretty new in the market place. What I like about this sweetener is that it is pretty low glycemic, at about 35, and most of its sugar is actually inulin. Inulin is a kind of sugar that the body does not actually metabolize, but instead the probiotic bacteria in our digestive tract consume the sugar as food, hence inulin is called a prebiotic. This makes coconut crystal a great option for a healthy sweetener.

Lastly, the whey protein provides protein, growth factors, and immune factors in a delicious and easy to digest form. Having this protein available to our muscles is crucial having sustained energy as well as a speedy recovery; also creating the irresistible, milky base that harbors longer-lasting sustainability.

Supreme Athletic Elixir Recipe

12 oz. Warm Gynostemma Tea
1 Tablespoon Coconut Oil
1 – 2 Tablespoons Coconut Crystals
2 Scoops Organic Whey Protein
1 tsp Polyrachis Extract
1 tsp Cordyceps Extract
1 tsp Astragalus Extract

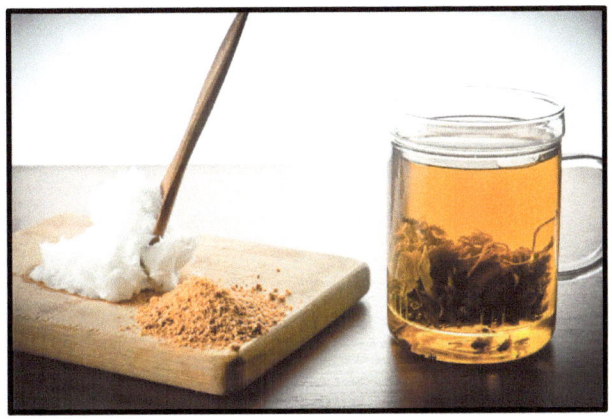

Directions

Add all ingredients to the blender and blend on high for about 60 seconds. Consume this elixir at your leisure.

Ultimate Natural High Elixir

The main superstars of this recipe are Phentlethyamine or "The Love Molecule," Anandaminde or "The Bliss Chemical", Dopamine, as well as various supportive nutrients, which can then keep these chemicals circulating and functioning longer.

What is Phenylethylamine(PEA)?

According to Wikipedia:

"Phenylethylamine is a natural monoamine alkaloid, trace amine, and also the name of a class of chemicals with many members well known for psychoactive drug and stimulant effects. Studies suggest that phenylethylamine functions as a neuromodulator or neurotransmitter in the mammalian central nervous system. Besides mammals, phenethylamine is found in many other organisms and foods such as chocolate. It is sold as a dietary supplement for purported mood and weight loss-related therapeutic benefits; however, orally ingested phenethylamine is usually inactive because of extensive first-pass metabolism by monoamine oxidase (MAO) into phenylacetic acid, preventing significant concentrations from reaching the brain."

PEA And The Theory Of Love

In the early 1980s, researcher Michael Liebowitz, author of the popular 1983 book The Chemistry of Love, remarked to reporters, "chocolate is loaded with PEA." This became the focus for an article in The New York Times, which was then taken up by the wire services, and then by magazine free-lancers, evolving into the now-eponymous "chocolate theory of love." However, as noted earlier, phenethylamine is rapidly metabolized by the enzyme MAO-B, preventing significant concentrations from reaching the brain, thus contributing no perceptible psychoactive effect without the use of a monoamine oxidase inhibitor (MAOI).

What does PEA do?

PEA has been dubbed "the love chemical" because it seems to uplift our mood while also helping to create feelings of attraction, excitement, and euphoria. PEA is noticeably abundant in the brains of happy people, whereas those whom are depressed will typically have lower levels of PEA. Some studies have shown that PEA can help to alleviate symptoms of depression with no side effects or chemical dependency.

The brain also releases PEA when we are sexually aroused with levels peaking at the orgasm. PEA also increases the activity of neurotransmitters in parts of the brain that control our ability to pay attention and stay alert. We naturally produce more PEA when we are fully engaged and captivated. In other words, I refer to the moments wherein we become so focused that we seem to lose all sense of time and even the outside world.

Another interesting thing is that when PEA is abundant the brain will pull in PEA in preference to dopamine, which then causes more dopamine to be active and available, thus raising our dopamine levels. Elevated dopamine levels are associated with enhanced concentration and a more positive mental outlook.

From this we can see that PEA is a chemical that mimics the brain chemistry of a person in love, thus elevating our mood while also helping us to have a better ability to have focus and sustained concentration.

The Superstars of The Ultimate Natural High Elixir

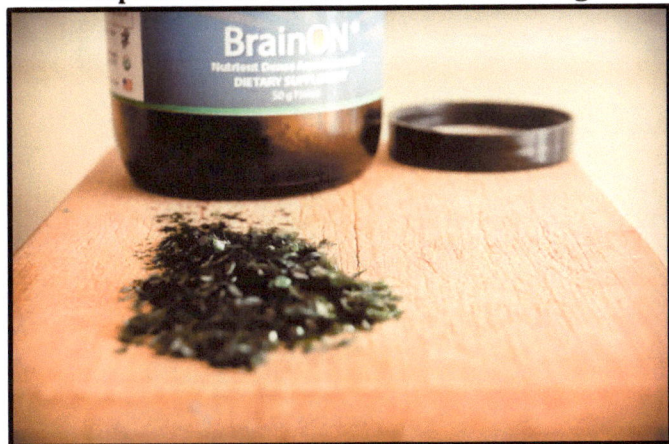

Now that we have gotten an introduction to PEA, let's take a look at some of the food sources of this chemical as well as the various supporting nutrients. Also, we will be illustrating the key players in this formula as well as exploring their unique chemistry.

The key players in this formula are: Raw Cacao, Blue Green Algae Extract, He Shou Wu Extract, and Mucuna Pruriens Extract.

What natural foods contain PEA?

The best natural sources of this chemical are Raw Cacao and Blue Green Algae. When purchasing the Cacao its best to get a raw product as heat processing destroys most of the active PEA. Also, while Blue Green Algae contains PEA, there are some products on the market that contain great concentrations, thus they are a better option when seeking out this unique chemical. My favorite of these options is E3Live's product, BrainOn.

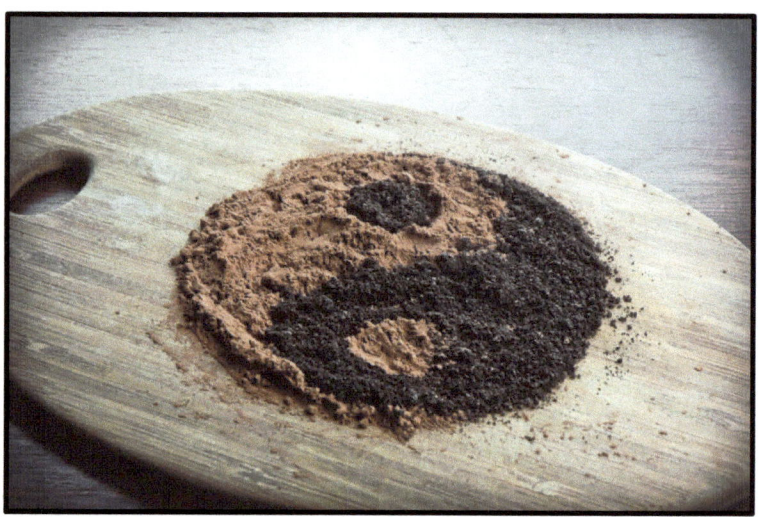

The Amazing Chemistry of Cacao

Raw cacao is very rich with essential minerals and antioxidants, but also very rich in rare chemicals that can positively affect our mood.

The first chemical is anadamide, which literally translated means "bliss chemical."

Findings from researchers at the Neurosciences Institute in San Diego, California indicate that "chocolate contains pharmacologically active substances that have the same effect on the brain as marijuana, but much, much, much weaker." Brain cells have a receptor for THC (tetrahydrocannabinol), which is the active ingredient in marijuana. A receptor is a structure on the surface of a cell that can lock onto certain molecules, making it possible to carry a signal through the cell wall. This means that active chemicals plug in like a key in a lock at various receptor sites. From this we can see that anandamide is the brain's own form of THC, as it works on the same pathways and plugs into the same receptor sites.

Anandamide, like other neurotransmitters, is broken down quickly after it's produced; yet cacao also contains chemicals that naturally slow down the breakdown of anadamide. This means that natural anandamide may stick around longer, making the positive effects last longer.

Cacao is also rich in the amino acid tryptophan, which is another powerful and mood enhancing nutrient This nutrient is essential for the production of our primary neurotransmitter, serotonin. Higher levels of serotonin are associated with diminished anxiety and a better ability to handle and process stress. Tryptophan also helps produce other neurotransmitters like melatonin and dimethyltryptamine.

In addition to being rich in PEA, anandamine, and tryptophan, cacao is one of the richest sources of magnesium, which is an essential mineral in the body that influences over 300 enzyme pathways, as well as our ability to stay relaxed and calm. Cacao also contains various types of neurotransmitter modulating agents, which allow serotonin and dopamine to remain in the bloodstream longer without being broken down. This means that not only does cacao contain chemicals that facilitate euphoria but it also the chemicals that help these feelings lost longer.

Blue Green Algae and PEA

Blue Green Algae is a rich source of phenylethylamine (PEA), which we have established as 'love molecule' because it increases the natural endorphins usually produced when we're in love or during exercise. PEA works by activating the neurotransmission of dopamine and other catecholamines in the brain. Unlike synthetic amphetamines, which are not easily metabolized and continue over-activating the nervous system to the point of damage, PEA is considered a natural neuro-modulator, which can be used according to our homeostatic needs and is quickly eliminated when it is no longer required. It is also a small molecule, which can easily pass through the intestinal membrane and the blood-brain barrier.

Once PEA is ingested, it is usually broken down by specific

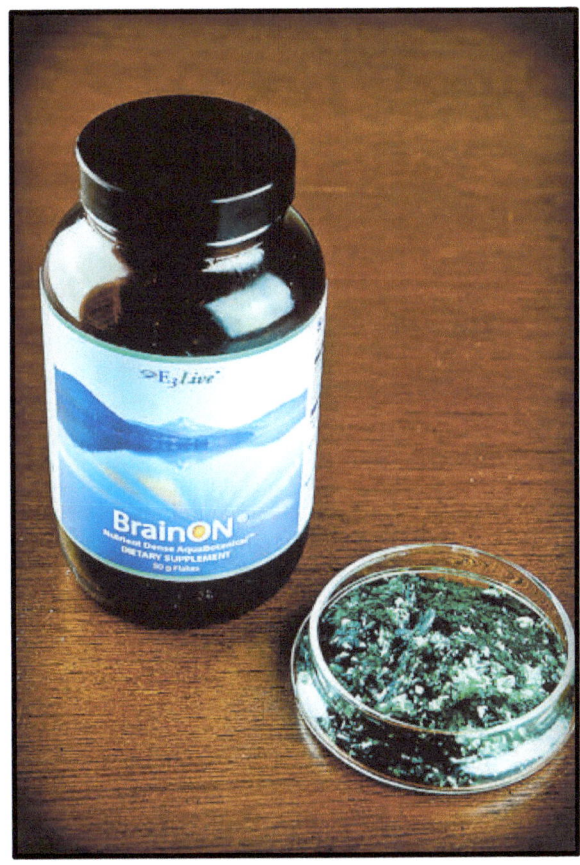

enzymes known as monoaminoxidase-B (or MAO-B), rendering it ineffective. But the PEA in Blue Green Algae is naturally protected from this phenomenon by powerful antioxidants. These function as natural MAO-B inhibitors, which protect the PEA allowing it to enter the brain to carry out its benefits. The MAO-B inhibitors have a similar inhibitory power comparable to that of the drug segeliline, used to treat Parkinson's disease, but without the side effects. The drug segeliline is an irreversible MAO-B inhibitor that destroys the enzymes, whilst natural inhibitors are reversible and only slow down their action.

Not only do these natural antioxidants – known as phycocyanins – protect the PEA, but they also provide a significant degree of neuro-protection. This is important because oxidative damage caused by emotional, nutritional and environmental stress is at the root of the progressive development of neurodegenerative conditions.

He Shou Wu and MAO-B

Researchers have found that of all herbs studied, he shou wu is the greatest inhibitor of MAO activity.

In animal studies, it was shown that he shou wu is very unique among plants as a **monoamine oxidase B inhibitor**. It specifically inhibits MAO-B activity, which is associated with the onset of geriatric senility. The primary benefit of MAO-B inhibition is an up-regulation of dopamine, which declines with age and is vital for mood, growth hormone release, sexual function, and coordination. After the age of 45 or 50, MAO-B activity increases significantly in the tissues of the brain. In one animal study, an MAO-B inhibition effect of over 80% was noted, suggesting that this is one of he shou wu's important anti-aging effects.

What we need to understand is that MAO is essentially an enzyme that breaks down dopamine. There are two types of MAO: "A" and "B." Some studies have shown that the two types of MAO activity appear to have different domains of activity in the body, whereas the brain has both types of activity. These two types of activity are mediated by different enzyme molecules and are regulated independently by endogenous and exogenous factors including genetic determinants, hormones, and aging. In humans, inhibition of MAO-A activity can lead to mood-enhancement. While having low levels of MAO-B has been associated with an increased susceptibility to mental imbalance and mental distress. This could be due to having low levels of dopamine caused because the body is recycling it to fast due to a shortage of MAO-B.

It's important to note that dopamine is a neurotransmitter associated with pleasure and well being that also helps to control the brain's reward and pleasure centers. Dopamine also helps regulate movement and emotional responses, and it enables us not only to see rewards, but also to take action to move toward them. So from this we can see how having low levels of this chemical can easily open the door for mental distress and imbalance.

From this brief example, we can see how in modern terms, the ancient claims made about he shou wu have been validated. We can also see why this is a great herb for helping to uplift the spirit by inhibiting monoamine oxidase B, which in turn can help us to have a greater amount of dopamine available in our system. Many authorities in the health field are now exploring avenues of combing he shou wu with other natural sources of neurotransmitters and chemicals that have positive effects on the mood and spirit.

The Rare and Unique Chemistry of Mucuna

Mucuna is famed for its rich concentration of L-DOPA, which is an amino acid that the body uses to produce dopamine, thus mucuna can naturally elevate our dopamine levels. Remember, dopamine is an important neurotransmitter, which plays a role in a wide range of brain functions. Dopamine affects movement, emotions, the experience of pleasure, and memory.

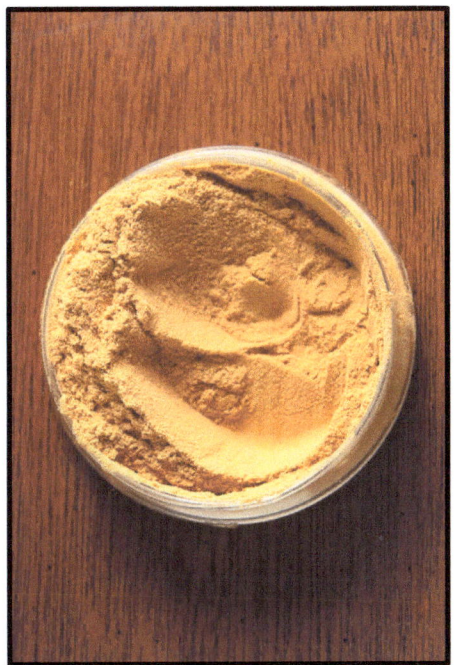

Insufficient levels of dopamine can lead to a wide range of serious symptoms, including:

- Depression;
- Inability to focus;
- Loss of motor control;
- Reduced sex drive;
- Cravings or addictions;
- Lack of motivation;
- Compulsions;
- Loss of pleasure or satisfaction.

People with low dopamine levels may experience feelings of depression, boredom, or apathy. They may lack the energy and motivation to carry out ordinary tasks, and they may have trouble focusing or making decisions.

In addition to L-DOPA, mucuna contains serotonin (5-HT), 5-HTP, nicotine, N,N-DMT (DMT), bufotenine, and 5-MeO-DMT.

The mature seeds of the plant contain about 3.1-6.1% L-DOPA, with trace amounts of 5-hydroxytryptamine (serotonin), nicotine, DMT-n-oxide, bufotenine, 5-MeO-DMT-n-oxide, and beta-carboline.

Bringing It All Together

As we saw earlier the key players in this formula are: Raw Cacao, Blue Green Algae Extract, He Shou Wu Extract, and Mucuna Pruriens Extract.

Now let us summarize and concisely understand how and why these ingredients synergize.

Raw Cacao
-Contains PEA
-Contains Anandamide
-Contains modulating agents which keep Anandamide in circulation longer
-Rich source of antioxidants to protect these delicate molecules
-Rich source of magnesium and other trace minerals that support relaxation and overall well-being
-Contains tryptophan, the precursor to serotonin, melatonin, and DMT

Blue Green Algae Extract BrainON
-Contains PEA
-Contains agents which keep PEA circulating longer
-Contains antioxidants to protect to delicate molecules
-Inhibits MAO

He Shou Wu Extract
-Inhibits MAO
-Rich source of zinc
-Rich source of antioxidants

Mucuna Pruriens Extract
-Contains L-DOPA
-Contains a wide array of other neurotransmitter modulating agents

So this all fits together as follows:

We get a rich source of the love, bliss, and pleasure chemicals from the Raw Cacao, BrainOn, and Mucuna Extract. These chemicals then combine with not only their own inherent MAO inhibiting properties, but also with the MAO inhibiting properties of He Shou Wu Extract. Remember that MAO is an enzyme which basically eats up our feel good chemicals so by inhibiting that enzyme, we are able to have more of these chemicals available. So basically what this means is that we get more noticeable, longer lasting effects.

Raw Cacao + BrainON + He Shou Wu Extract + Mucuna Extract = A rich concentration of feel good pleasure chemicals as well as the necessary co-factors to make these bio-available while also increasing the potency and duration of their effects.

Ultimate Natural High Elixir Recipe

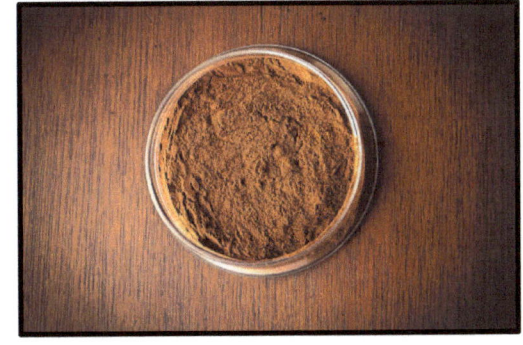

12 oz. Warm Gynostemma Tea
1 Tablespoon Coconut Oil
1 -2 Tablespoons Coconut Crystals
2 Tablespoons Raw Cacao Powder
1 tsp BrainON Powder
1 -2 tsp He Shou Wu Extract
1 -2 tsp Mucuna Pruriens Extract

Directions

Add all ingredients to the blender and blend on high for about 60 seconds. Consume this elixir at your leisure.

Bone Marrow Jing Builder

This recipe is a deep and profound collection of herbs to support and nourish the jing energy. Jing can be thought of as our deep stores of energy, our hormonal reserves, as well as our sexual potency. Jing is also heavily associated with the bones and the bone marrow. In my mind, Cordyceps and Polyrachis are two of the most powerful and well-tolerated jing tonics. Both of these herbs contain and nourish both the yin and yang aspects of the kidney jing energy, which is partially what makes them so well tolerated by most people.

Cordyceps has been shown in studies to be protective to the bone marrow while also enhancing the maturation and proliferation of bone marrow cells. In China, Cordyceps is also regarded as one of the top longevity and rejuvenation tonics. It is used by healthy people to maintain, promote, and lengthen life, and used by sick people or those in a weakened state to regain lost energy and vitality. From these polar examples we can see why cordyceps is such an alley for this recipe.

The phycocyanin from Blue Majik has also been shown in studies to enhance the proliferation and differentiation of bone marrow cells. For this reason there are a few high priced products that aim to aid in stem cell regeneration and feature this extract as the main ingredient. These kinds of products are used to support the bodys natural renewal system by supporting the release of more stem cells into the blood stream, which then help the body to maintain and repair tissue and organs. If we were to look for a modern corollary to the Chinese concept of jing, I believe this is a top candidate.

Jing is thought to be the energy, which determines the quality and quantity of our life. Obviously, if we are wanting to have a long, high quality life, then on a bio-physical level we will need a sufficient level of stem cells to keep our tissue and organs repaired and regenerated. This is what the synergy of this elixir aims to accomplish at a fraction of the cost of the other products on the market.

Bone Marrow Jing Building Recipe

12 oz. Warm Gynostemma Tea
1 Tablespoon Coconut Oil
1 -2 Scoops Organic Whey Protein
1 -2 Tablespoons Coconut Crystals
1 -2 Tablespoons Raw Cacao Powder
1/2 tsp Blue Majik Powder
1 tsp Polyrachis Extract
1 tsp Cordyceps Extract

Directions

Add all ingredients to the blender and blend on high for about 60 seconds. Consume this elixir at your leisure.

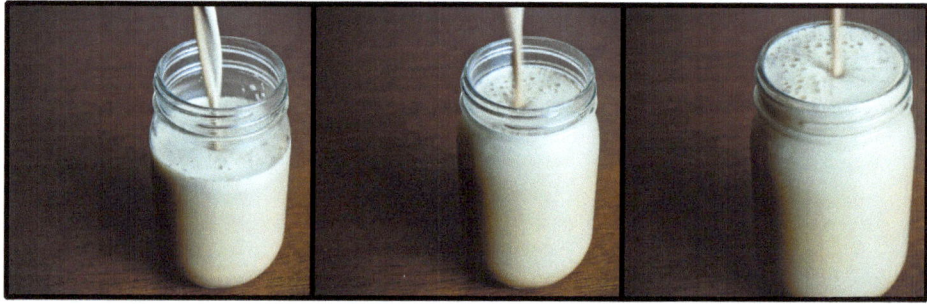

Invincible Immunity Elixir

The elixir combines the most powerful nutrients for the immune system in a synergistic, delicious, and potent blend that deeply nourishes the immune system.

The main super stars of this elixir are Gynostemma, Duanwood Reishi, Cordyceps, Colostrum, Camu, and Blue Majik.

Gynostemma, Reishi, and Cordyceps typically have a kind of bitter earthly flavor and this is mostly due to their rich concentration of triterpenes and polysaccharides.

Triterpenes are a group of active natural compounds found in most plants. As with most beneficial substances in plants, it protects the plant from microbial infection. However, in the human body triterpenes are believed to strengthen digestion, improve allergies, and fight inflammation.

The triterpenes found in these herbs are thought to play various important roles for the well being of human body by being antifungal, antibacterial, and antiviral. These triterpenes also helps to improve high blood pressure and balance blood lipids. Some studies have also shown that these chemicals are involved in transmitting nerve impulses to the brain's cortex and thus can aid in enhancing all central nervous system functions. These chemicals are also thought to modulate the action of hormones and maintain stability among various body systems.

A polysaccharide is basically a long chain sugar molecule, which is unique for a couple of reasons. First, it is bitter in taste due to its long chain chemical structure, unlike other sugars like fructose or sucrose, which are very sweet to the taste and have a very limited action in the body with their very short chain chemical structure. These polysaccharides are also unique because they plug into receptor sites on immune cells, a process which helps the immune system to do its job more effectively and efficiently. It is important to note that this is not an immune stimulant or immune depressant effect but more so immuno-regulation or balancing.

These herbs do not simply stimulate or depress the immune system like many other immuno-influencing herbs. In fact, they actually balance and modulate the immune system, or in the other words, assist the immune system where it needs assisting. For instance, if there is an area, which is under active, it can bring it back up to balance. If there is an area that is over active, it can actually tone that down to balance. This indicates that these herbs are very intelligent and worthy of the title 'adaptogens' because they not only help us adapt to stress, but they also intelligently and gently adapt to the current level of homeostasis in the body. One of the most profound qualities of adaptogens is that it is physically impossible to replicate their adaptive function in any conventional medicine. Their bidirectional intelligence can be matched by nothing man-made.

This is beneficial and important for a myriad of reasons. One of them being the fact that virus and bacteria are intelligent organisms, which are constantly evolving and changing. Keeping this in mind, it might make sense to ingest things that's are able to keep our immune system strong and balanced. Secondly, we are constantly being exposed to stressors and toxins in our environment, which can have negative effects on our immune system. The daily experience of living can even stress us out through which we can now understand the effects that the stress hormones like cortisol can have on the immune system.

From these very few examples, perhaps you can now see and understand the importance of consuming immuno-regulating herbs on a regular basis; Herbs, which are adaptogens and intelligent, not merely immune stimulants or immune depressants, but herbs, which gently balance, modulate, and strengthen over time and in accordance to the needs of our bodies.

Colostrum is the "immune milk" produced by all mammals for only the first few hours before and after birth. It contains an astounding 97 immune factors and 87 growth factors, which have been known to enhance rejuvenation and regeneration while strengthening the immune system. These immune factors essentially provide the immune system with information on how to handle certain pathogens, thus educating your immune system and enhancing its protective abilities.

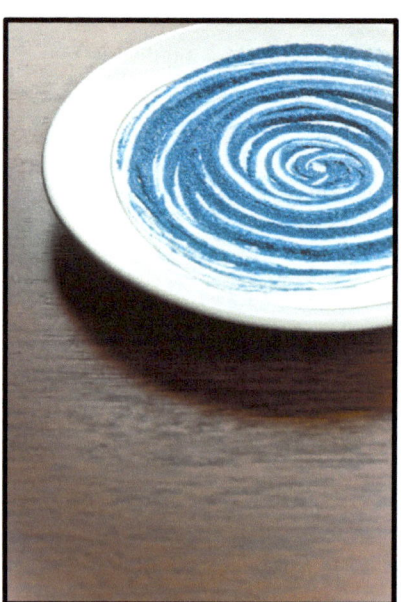

Camu camu has more Vitamin C than any other known plant in the world. This allows it to deeply support the immune system while also potentiating the actions and efficacy of the other ingredients in this elixir. This fruit has also been known to promote healthy gums, eyes and skin while improve mood and mental functions.

Blue Majik is an extract of Arthrospira platensis, nutrient dense algae. It is made up primarily of Phycocyanin, a powerful antioxidant that can quench free radicals and has been shown to be a potent natural COX-2 inhibitor. The Phycocyanin level is greater than 30% in this product. What this equates to is: a minimum of 300mg of Phycocyanin per 1 gram of product. Based on research, Phycocyanin is a super nutrient for the immune system. Studies have found that it helps to stimulate production of bone marrow and stem cells, which thereby enhance the proliferation of various immune cells. Phycocyanin also helps support Super Oxide Dismutase and other endogenous enzymes in the body with assist in cleansing and detoxification.

This is an extremely powerful combination, synergizing and supplementing itself. The herbs form a base of immune modulation, which can strengthen, and balance the immune system. The colostrum provides all the known growth and immune factors, which can inform and educate the immune system. The camu potentiates the actions of these ingredients while also boosting the immune system, and lastly, the Blue Majik potentiates all of the ingredients by stimulating bone marrow and stem cell production, while also enhancing cellular detoxification.

Invincible Immunity Elixir Recipe

12 oz. Warm Gynostemma Tea
1 Tablespoon Coconut Oil
1 -2 Tablespoons Coconut Crystals
1 -2 Tablespoons Raw Cacao Powder(Optional)
1 -2 Tablespoons Colostrum Powder
1/4 – 1/2 tsp Camu Camu Powder
1/4 - 1/2 tsp Blue Majik Powder
1 tsp Duanwood Reishi Extract
1 tsp Cordyceps Extract

Directions

Add all ingredients to the blender and blend on high for about 60 seconds. Consume this elixir at your leisure. Feel free to add a flavor of your choice to take the elixir to the next level. This could be 1 -2 Tablespoons of Cacao powder, a handful of berries, etc.

Relaxation Manifestation Elixir

This is really where it all started for me and, for that reason, this recipe is near and dear to my heart. There is something so nourishing and warming about the simple combination of reishi and he shou wu. Reishi is, of course, the mushroom of immortality and the herb of spiritual potency. He Shou Wu is one of the most famous anti-aging and longevity herbs. Together their relaxation effects seem to be amplified and accentuated in a way that I can describe as feeling grounded, centered, calm, and strong. Feel free to consume this one whenever you feel the need to relax and let go of stress. Taken at night, both herbs can help facilitate a deep and restful sleep.

Relaxation Manifestation Elixir Recipe

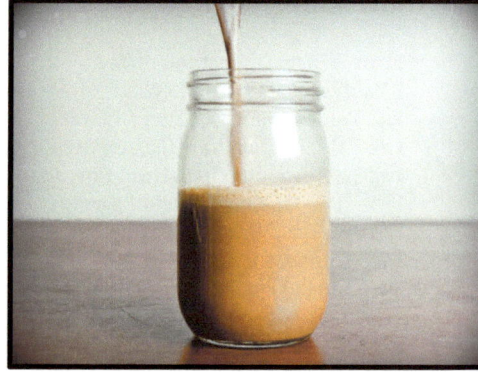

12 oz. Warm Gynostemma Tea
1 Tablespoon Coconut Oil
1 -2 Tablespoons Coconut Crystals
1 -2 Scoops Organic Whey Protein
1/4 tsp Vanilla Powder
1 tsp He Shou Wu Extract
1 tsp Reishi Extract
Optional: 1 TB Cacao Powder or Dandy Blend

Directions

Add all ingredients to the blender and blend on high for about 60 seconds. Consume this elixir at your leisure.

60 Second Gallbladder Cleanse

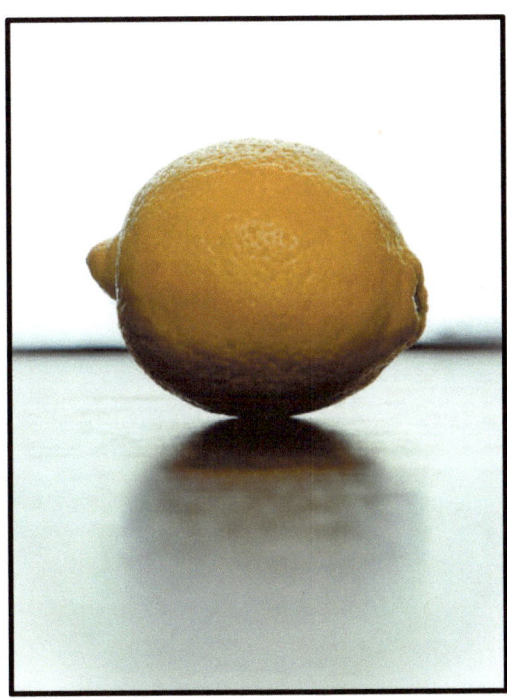

First thing in the morning and on an empty stomach, consume the juice of half a lemon in 8 ounces of warm/hot water. Simply take 8 ounces of spring water and heat it up on the stove. Bring it up to the temperate of tea or coffee, and remove from the stove. Then, add the juice of half a lemon and consume. This combination of lemon juice and hot water done first in thing in the morning will stimulate and cleanse your liver and gallbladder. This recipe is very simple and quick, while also being extremely potent and effective. The combo also works great if you've been partying or drinking too much, didn't eat well the night before, generally feeling sluggish and backed up, or as a daily dose of vitamin C.

60 Second ProBiotic Cleanse

This recipe is a great way to quickly colonize the digestive tract with billions of beneficial bacteria that will help to clean the blood, detox the digestive tract, as well as enhance the cognitive functions. Keep in mind, we are actually 10x more bacteria than we are human cells, so the level of our probiotics is a crucial and foundational element for our health and vitality. It's also a great way to quickly and easily clean out the system, hence the title, 60 Second Probiotic Cleanse.

This recipe is very simple and requires only two ingredients and one step in thinking outside "the box". The ingredient is an entire bottle of probiotics and the second is about 8 ounces of kombucha, coconut water kefir, or water kefir, whichever is most accessible. Now, please keep in mind this is something you want to definitely do on an empty stomach and at night an hour or two before bed. Also, make sure you have some time to be around a toilet the next morning. The first time you do this, you may experience some gas and extra elimination. After the first or second time these symptoms will dissipate as your over all gut health and level of beneficial bacteria reaches a higher level of homeostasis. The probiotics or good bacteria pushing out and replacing opportunistic bacteria, toxins, undigested foods, and general stagnation are the likely cause the gas and elimination. Keep in mind this is a temporary process and will 'pass' with time.

This is a great one to do once every few months, or as you intuitive feel. It's also great to do before or after traveling to really reset, cleanse, and build up the level of probiotics. This is typically when I use this strategy; otherwise I just pay attention to my gut and how it's feeling. If I feel off in the digestive system or if it seems like a good idea to do, I generally just follow that. This strategy, in combination with the regular consumption of cultured foods, can do a lot to restore gut health, which in turn boosts the immune system, detoxes the body, as well as improving cognitive functions.

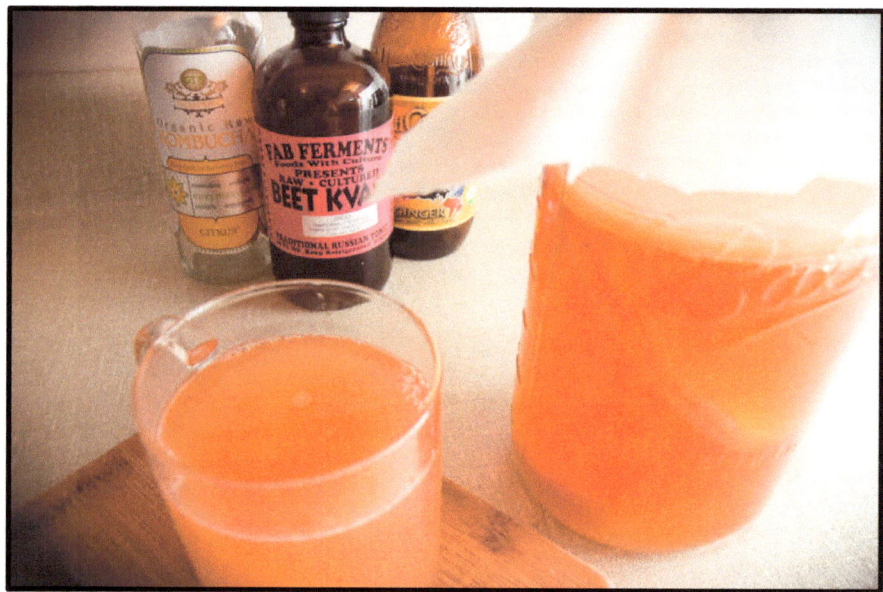

Two questions may ensure from reading about this seemingly radical cleanse. The first being, is this safe, and the second being, what kind of probiotics should I get. To answer the first question, yes this is a safe practice. I've been doing this for years, as have many of my friends and clients. These probiotics are amazing for what they can do in the body and if you are new to the subject I highly encourage you to do more research. Its also important to note that we are actually 10x more bacteria than we are human cells, so wouldn't it make sense to do our best to make sure we are made up the right kinds of bacteria? There is literally no way to overdose on bacteria, whether in one consumption or overtime.

To answer the second question I will share with you what I generally do. I use a couple of criteria when I decide which bottle of probiotics to go for. The first criteria is whatever is available at the local health food store or Vitamin Shoppe and the second criteria is how much I feel like spending at that moment in time. Typically, I stick with the $30 to $35 range and from there I go with the available product which as the highest levels of probiotics. In the past I have used brands such as RenewLife, DDS, and Garden of Life, all of which have been pretty successful. Some other probiotics can reach higher prices or be more specific to your age or gender, but I generally just stick with the highest levels of bacteria and maximum strength formulas. If you have any questions beyond that, I would consult the vendor at your retail location.

So, hopefully that has answered your questions and given you a good working model to ease your transition from being liberated from directions and labels. Now, let's explain the actual procedure for what we'll do for this recipe.

First, you want to make sure you have a bottle of a cultured beverage. Again, this could be kombucha, coconut water kefir, or water kefir, all of which are available at your local health food store or you can make at home.

Secondly, you want to make sure you have a bottle of probiotics that you feel good about.

The third step in the process is opening the bottle of probiotics and consuming the entire thing with your cultured beverage of choice. It's worth mentioning here that if you are nervous, short of funds, or have a hard time swallowing capsules, then feel free to consume half the bottle now and then the other half at a later date. That is no problem, always listen to your gut and feel out the best option.

The reason we want to consume the probiotics with a cultured beverage is that the beverage is also loaded with probiotics and enzymes, which will assist and facilitate the digestion and assimilation of the probiotics from the bottle. The two together form a great alliance that creates a synergistic and thus enhanced effect.

5 Elements Elixir

Schizandra is one of the true heroes of tonic herbalism, due to its rare attribute of having all five flavors and thus nourishing all five organs.

Properties of Schizandra:

- Prolongevity
- Balancing adaptogen
- Optimizes beauty and skin
- Sharpens mind and improves coordination and memory
- Improves sexual function, endurance and performance
- Tonifies the kidney and liver
- Rejuvenates and restores respiratory functionality, power and circulation
- Purifies blood
- Powerful cleansing and detoxification properties
- Contains all 5 tastes, 5 elements, 12 meridians and 3 treasures

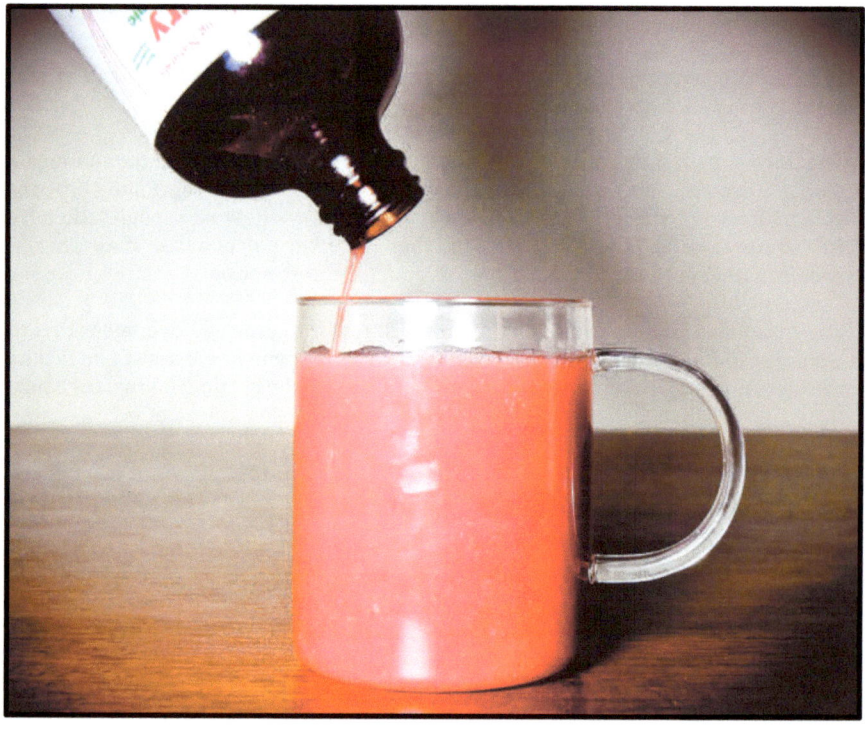

Named by the Chinese, "Wu Wei Zi", directly translated as "Five Taste Fruit," Schizandra not only embodies all five tastes, sour, bitter, sweet, pungent and salty, but in the same respect, resonates with all five elements, while infiltrating all twelve meridians and offering its gifts from all three treasures, Jing, Qi and Shen. Staying true to its form, Schizandra integrates with the human body in the same light, scoring ten's across the board. You name it, Schizandra helps it, and ranking as one of the most renowned adaptogens on the planet, its primary focus is balance, as there is no limit to the amount or frequency of intake. In fact, the best way to get the most out of your Schizandra, or any adaptogen for that matter, is maintaining intake for prolonged time periods, as "homeostasis" is Schizandra's ultimate long-term goal for you.

Revered since as early as 2000 B.C. in ancient Chinese history as a quintessential herbal substance, Schizandra Berry has not only been used regularly by Chinese royalty, but has ranked highly in many herbal honors. Throughout history, its primary uses have been focused around beauty and sex, pictured in ancient art as a symbol of longevity and immortality. Exalted as one of the most powerful "youth tonics" of all time, Schizandra has held true to its reputation, rejuvenating skin, helping to maintain its moisture while also protecting it from outside stressors. With usage overtime, it has also been proven to reduce and protect from wrinkles. The powerful astringent properties of Schizandra Berry places it right on top of the line, ahead of all natural or expensive beauty care products- and its pretty much the most delicious and dynamic tasting herb known to existence. To address the sex end of the herb lightly (and I mean very lightly), Schizandra enhances drive in both men and women, for men improving sexual function and endurance, and in woman, increasing water qi from the kidney (and other areas) while counter-acting vaginal discharge. As Schizandra also has been said to be a powerful aphrodisiac, this herb may optimize your love life beyond explored territory.

Reaching beyond the surface, Schizandra berry dives deep into your system, circulating its goodness throughout your entire body and working systems (literally). It strengthens your respiratory system and purifies your blood, as it increases circulation. Schizandra opens up the airways, allowing all this purified blood and oxygen travel throughout each of your organs, even reaching those dark and dusty corners that got sore after your neglected them for so many years. Naturally, this increased oxygen flow runs straight into your brain, making Schizandra an extremely effective mind tonic. Acting as a mock-nootropic, this herb increases alertness without a stimulant effect- a wakeful focus. While also known to have a calming effect, you can have the best of both worlds. As though it wasn't working hard enough, Schizandra is also a tenacious anti-oxidant, with cleansing properties ranking with Reishi. Your liver will thank you. Among its other unmentioned amazing qualities are balancing your nervous system, refining coordination, improving memory, enhancing vision, increasing sensitivity and strengthening endurance.

By combining Schizandra with the cultured beverage kombucha, you can further enhance and potentiate the effects it can have. This is because kombucha is also sour, especially if using the citrus flavor. This sour flavor is known to nourish and stimulate the liver. Also kombucha is rich with enzymes and probiotics, which can synergize and enhance the Schizandra. On top of that, it is just a purely delicious and delightful combination.

5 Elements Elixir Recipe

8 oz. Citrus Kombucha
2 – 4 oz. Schizandra Juice

Directions

Pour the kombucha into your glass and then add your desired about of Schizandra juice. Give the glass a quick stir or swirl and consume as your leisure

Mile High Blue Majik Chai

This recipe is aptly titled because after consuming it, you may feel a mile high. And well, the color of the drink will be a blue-greenish color. The combination of Blue Majik and BrainOn powder is truly a unique and magical pairing. These algae extracts have been shown to be massively anti-inflammatory, immune modulating, and mood uplifting. They are also deeply nourishing, given their concentration of vitamins, minerals, essential fatty acids, and psychoactive compounds. In my eyes, this elixir is a modern marvel and worthy of being a wonder of the world. I say this because we are so fortunate to have access to these powerful substances. Never before in history have these substances been so easily accessible and, likewise, been so easily combined in such a delicious and potent manner.

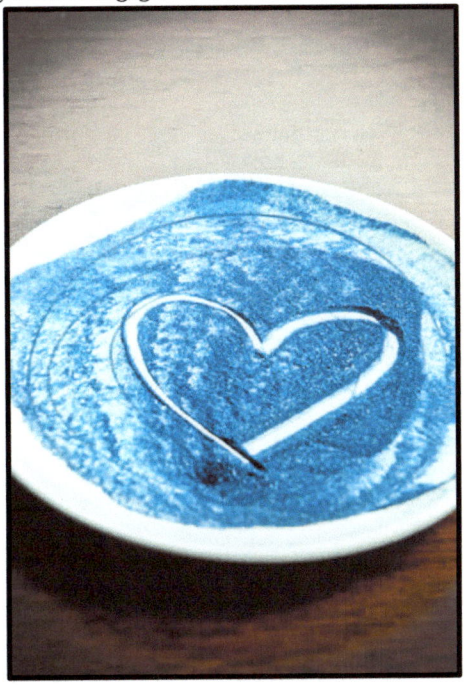

Mile High Blue Majik Chai Recipe

12 oz. Warm Gynostemma Tea
1 Tablespoon Coconut Oil
1 -2 Tablespoons Coconut Crystals
1 -2 Scoops Organic Whey Protein
1/4 - 1/2 tsp Blue Majik Powder
1/4 – 1/2 tsp BrainOn Powder
1/4 tsp Vanilla Powder
1 Tablespoon Chai Spice Mix

Directions

Add all ingredients to the blender and blend on high for about 60 seconds. Consume this elixir at your leisure.

10 Second NutMilk Recipe

Never again will you have to worry about buying nutmilk at the store or spending a long time making your own. This recipe requires just a few simple ingredients, taking mere seconds to prepare, and is far cheaper than anything you can buy at the store.

10 Second NutMilk

12 oz. Gynostemma Tea or 12 oz. Spring Water
2 Tablespoons Raw Organic Hemp Seeds
1 -2 Tablespoons Coconut Crystals
1/4 tsp Vanilla Powder
Pinch of Celtic Sea Salt or Himalayan Salt

Directions

Add all ingredients to the blender and blend for 30 – 60 seconds. The milk is ready to consume as is. You can also use it as a base for other elixirs or even pour over cereal or granola.

Liver Cleansing Tea

This recipe combines two of the best herbs for stimulating cleanse and detoxification of the liver/gallbladder. Both herbs are known to be digestive aids, mild diuretics, mild laxatives, and blood purifiers. For this reason, we can see that they are obviously not tonic herbs, and thus should not be consumed over the long term. Long meaning, every day for months, or even years, like a tonic adaptogen should or could be in consuming. That's an important difference to keep in mind here. There are different classes of herbs, some are more medicinal, and thus less ideal for long term, and some are more like foods and more well suited for long-term regular consumption.

I like to use this simple tea formula usually around springtime when it feels right to get the liver energy moving. In Chinese Medicine, the liver is associated with the season of spring, thus it makes sense to support the liver at this time. That being said, I also use this tea anytime I am feeling sluggish or heavy, as this tea really helps to get things moving in the digestive tract. Also, the liver has a profound effect on the emotions and the nervous system so this tea can sometimes stir up suppressed emotions.

The flavor of this tea is generally pretty bitter and earthy, so please don't be afraid of this. Learning to enjoy the bitter flavor is one of the best things a person can do for their health. These days we are too focused on sweet, sometimes salty, and sometimes spicy, but generally, never bitter. This is obviously unbalancing and, thus, can negatively affect our health.

Liver Cleansing Tea Recipe

16 oz. Spring Water
2 Tablespoons Dandelion Root
1 Tablespoon Yellow Dock Root

Directions

Add all ingredients to a pot on the stove and bring the water just up to a boil. From there reduce to medium heat and simmer for 30 – 60 minutes. Strain off the herbs and tea is ready to consume. Also, you can re-cook these herbs 3 times.

Consume tea as is if you prefer a bitter brew. If you prefer something more pleasurable please see the Liver Cleansing Elixir Recipe.

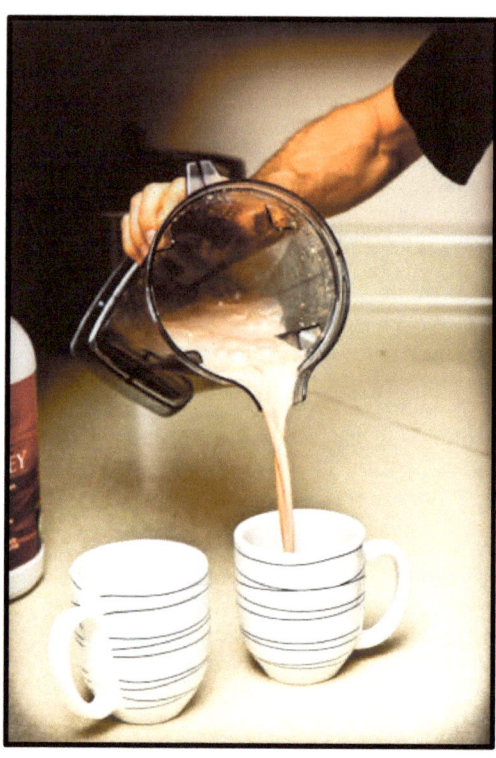

Liver Cleansing Elixir Recipe

Since the tea itself it rather bitter, I like to use this simple recipe to dress it up a bit and turn it into more of a delicious and sustainable elixir. If you are just wanting something light, then just stick with the tea, but if you'd like something more tasty and nourishing then this is the recipe for you.

12 oz. Warm Liver Cleansing Tea
1 Tablespoon Coconut Oil
1 -2 Tablespoons Coconut Crystals
1 -2 Scoops Organic Whey Protein
1/4 tsp Vanilla Powder
2 tsp Chai Spice Mix
Yerba Prima Liquid Bentonite Clay

Directions

Add all ingredients to the blender and blend on high for about 60 seconds. Consume this elixir at your leisure.

After consuming this elixir, wait about 10 or 15 minutes then consume 1 Tablespoon of liquid bentonite clay. Be sure to pay attention to your water intake through the rest of the day, as it's a good idea to drink more water when consuming clay. When you consume bentonite, it expands and forms into gel and which helps to remove toxins from the body. It absorbs things such as free radicals, harmful bacteria, pesticides, and heavy metals. When it enters into the intestine, it also has the capacity to absorb waste item from the intestine walls and remove it completely from our body. This works to our advantage because we are stimulating our liver and gallbladder with the Liver Cleansing Tea, so we want to make sure that everything our liver is processing and eliminating is easily and safely neutralized and eliminated. This is what the clay functions to do in this instance, basically the gel forms and soaks up the things the liver and gallbladder are removing. By absorbing toxins before they enter the bloodstream, clay reduces the overload of toxins that the liver and kidneys normally have to filter out again. By eliminating the buildup of waste lodged in the lower colon, clay also allows the body to absorb more nutrients, vitamins and minerals.

How To Make Your Own Chai Spice Mix

Having your own chai spice blend is a great way to transform a simple elixir into something extraordinary and extremely delicious.

It's important to keep in mind that this recipe is versatile and customizable and should always be made to your taste. Some may like it a bit sweeter while others may prefer a spicier chai, this is entirely up to you.

To begin you will need some or all of the following powdered herbs:

Cinnamon
Ginger
Cloves
Cardamom
Black Pepper

For my taste I like to have cinnamon and ginger be the most dominant flavors and then have the cloves, cardamom, and black pepper serve as supportive notes.

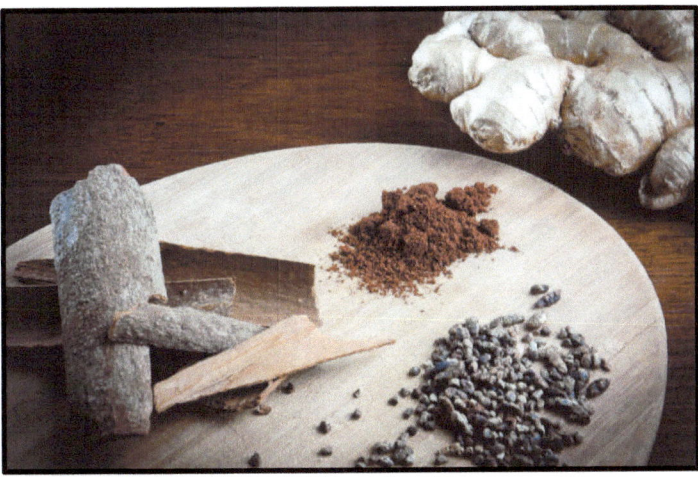

Here are the ratios I like to use:

1 TB Cinnamon
1 tsp Ginger
1/4 tsp cloves
1/4 tsp cardamom
1/8 tsp black pepper

Optional:
2 tsp Coconut Sugar
Pinch of Salt
Pinch of Cayenne Pepper

Again, keep in mind this is what tastes good to me, while you may like something different. A good principle is to start off with is using less of the more potent spices and gradually adding more while tasting as you go along. Eventually, you will find a ratio that you enjoy and that works well for you. The next time around you will have a solid basis from which to build your own personalized chai spice mix.

The procedure here is actually quite simple. Start off with a plastic bag or small glass jar of your choice. Then simply add your powders and shake/stir. From here, dip your finger in and give your mix a taste to see if it's where you want it to be. If not, then add a bit more until you find an enjoyable mix. Again, start with less and you can always add more.

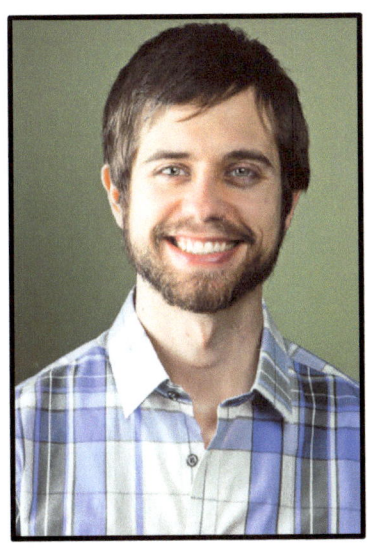

A Note in Closing

This is a precious diamond that has been produced from the layers upon layers of research and experience, both personally and professionally tested to be effective and quite delicious! My hope is to have given you a vast understanding of how delicate the cohesion of a great-tasting, metabolically inclined elixir can be. You now have a solid foundation to fully embrace the world of elixir crafting. Using these basic rules and recipes to customize drinks to your tastes and metabolism, you are now able to explore the profound depths of elixirs, setting the stage for the transformative health upgrades that follow you along this path.

Resources

Tonic Herbs:
Astragalus Extract - http://hyperionherbs.com
Cordyceps Extract - http://hyperionherbs.com
He Shou Wu Extract - http://hyperionherbs.com
Mucuna Extract - http://hyperionherbs.com
Polyrachis Extract - http://hyperionherbs.com
Reishi Extract - http://hyperionherbs.com
Gynostemma Tea - http://hyperionherbs.com

Magikal Blue Powders:
BrainOn Powder – http://hyperionherbs.com
Blue Majik Powder – http://hyperionherbs.com

Flavors:
Cacao Powder - http://ultimatesuperfoods.com
Vanilla Powder - http://ultimatesuperfoods.com
DandyBlend - http://amazon.com
Frozen Berries - Your local health food store

Chai Mix:
Cinnamon - http://bit.ly/chiachia
Ginger - http://bit.ly/gherbspage

Cloves - http://bit.ly/chiachia
Cardamom - http://bit.ly/chiachia
Black Pepper - http://bit.ly/bherbspage

Protein Powders:
Organic Grass Fed Whey Protein - http://hyperionherbs.com
Rice Protein - http://amazon.com
Hemp Protein - http://amazon.com

Oils:
Coconut Oil - http://bit.ly/cheapcoconutoil
Ghee - http://www.pureindianfoods.com/
Raw Organic Butter – Your local farmer or farmers market
Cacao Butter - http://ultimatesuperfoods.com

Soluble Fibers:
Chia Seeds - http://bit.ly/chiachia
Irish Moss – http://amazon.com
Slippery Elm Bark - http://bit.ly/slipslipelmelm

Sweeteners:
You can easily find these are your local health food store
Coconut Crystals
Raw Honey
Raw Agave
Stevia

Water:
Fresh Spring Water – http://findaspring.com

Other:
Dandelion - http://bitly/dherbspage
Yellow dock - http://bit.ly/yherbspage
You can find the following at your local health food store:
Bentonite Clay - Yerba Prima Bentonite Clay
Kombucha Tea (raw, unpasteurized)
Probiotics

www.ingramcontent.com/pod-product-compliance
Lightning Source LLC
Chambersburg PA
CBHW050832290526
45792CB00001B/358